They Say You're Crazy

Paula J. Caplan, Ph.D.

THEY
SAY
YOU'RE
CRAZY

How the World's
Most Powerful Psychiatrists
Decide Who's Normal

Addison-Wesley Publishing Company
Reading, Massachusetts   Menlo Park, California   New York
Don Mills, Ontario   Wokingham, England   Amsterdam   Bonn
Sydney   Singapore   Tokyo   Madrid   San Juan
Paris   Seoul   Milan   Mexico City   Taipei

Many of the designations used by manufacturers and sellers to distinguish their products are claimed as trademarks. Where those designations appear in this book and Addison-Wesley was aware of a trademark claim, the designations have been printed in initial capital letters (e.g., Maalox).

Library of Congress Cataloging-in-Publication Data

Caplan, Paula J.
    They say you're crazy : how the world's most powerful
psychiatrists decide who's normal / by Paula J. Caplan.
      p.   cm.
    Includes bibliographical references and index.
    ISBN 0-201-40758-2
    ISBN 0-201-48832-9 (pbk.)
    1. Diagnostic and Statistical Manual of Mental Disorders.
2. Mental illness—Classification—Political aspects. 3. Mental
illness—Classification—Social aspects. 4. Mental illness—
Diagnosis—Political aspects. 5. Mental illness—Diagnosis—Social
aspects.   I. Title.
RC455.2.C4C37   1995
616.89—dc20   94-39662
                                              CIP

Cover design by Jean Seal
Text design by Edith Allard
Set in 11-point Janson by Jackson Typesetting Co., Jackson, MI

1 2 3 4 5 6 7 8 9-DOH-0099989796
First printing, March 1995
First paperback printing, February 1996

For Graham, with love

Reading about the evolution of the DSM, to its third revised
power, is somewhat like reading the history of the Balkans:
ongoing border wars, eruptions, skirmishes, the odd assassina-
tion, uprising, overthrow. . . .

To read about the evolution of the DSM is to know this:
It is an entirely political *document. What it includes, what*
it does not include, are the result of intensive campaigning,
lengthy negotiating, infighting, and power plays.

—*Louise Armstrong*
And They Call It Help:
The Psychiatric Policing of America's Children

Contents

Acknowledgments

My deepest appreciation goes to my parents, Tac Karchmer Caplan and Jerry Caplan, for their constant, loving support of my work all these years and for specific suggestions about the content of this book. Thanks to Mom also for saying she wanted me to "let" her read my work as it progressed, just when I was assuming it would be an imposition to ask her to read it. Thanks to Dad also for sending me treasure troves of clippings, most of which end up somehow in what I write. I want also to say how much I appreciate the support of my precious, now-grown children, Jeremy Benjamin Caplan and Emily Julia Caplan.

My gratitude also goes to former *Canadian Psychology/ Psychologie canadienne* editor Pat O'Neill, for inviting me to write the article which became the seed for this book; to Lenore Walker for moral and practical support at the book proposal stage; to Jeffrey Moussaieff Masson, for introducing me to my wonderful editor, Nancy Miller; to Nancy Miller, for all her thoughtful and detailed suggestions and encouragement; to Paul Mohl, for reminding me of how long-standing has been my interest in this subject; to Donna Sharon and Jim Williams, for sharing their thoughts about an early draft of chapter 1; to June Larkin,

Kaye-Lee Pantony, Maureen Gans, and Joan McCurdy-Myers, for coauthoring with me some key papers on which I have drawn extensively for this book; to Mary Brown Parlee, Lianne Yoshida, Bonnie Bean, Elaine Borins, Dianne Corlett, Marlene Levitt, Mara Milakovic, Kathryn Morgan, Cleta Moyer, Monica Piebrock, and Cecilia Settino for their help in organizing the campaign against classifying premenstrual syndrome as a psychiatric disorder; to Brydon Gombay, Carol Landau, and Lynn Marcus for providing helpful articles and books; to Janet Surrey and Steve Bergman for their encouraging feedback about the manuscript; to Terrence McNally for thinking of the title, *They Say You're Crazy*; to Mark Salzer, for help in the Brown University computer center; and to Graham Berman, for having taught me so much and been so encouraging over the years, for listening to the beginnings of the ideas for this book, and for giving me deeply thoughtful feedback on drafts and discussion about many of the issues and the approach.

Preface

I have written this book with a very limited purpose in mind: to help people see how decisions are made about who is normal. I believe that knowing how such decisions are made can help a person overcome the damage that is done to so many who are called—or who consider themselves—abnormal. As a clinical and research psychologist who for some years worked as a psychotherapist, I have seen a great many people who have suffered such harm. As a former consultant to those who construct the world's most influential manual of alleged mental illness, the American Psychiatric Association's (APA) *Diagnostic and Statistical Manual of Mental Disorders* (*DSM*), I have had an insider's look at the process by which decisions about abnormality are made. As a longtime specialist in teaching and writing about research methods, I have been able to assess and monitor the truly astonishing extent to which scientific methods and evidence are disregarded as the handbook is being developed and revised.

I have made no attempt to document the long, horrific history of mistreatments and misdiagnoses by mental health professionals of all kinds, since others have done so in remarkable books. Mistreatment is an almost inevitable result of diagnosis that is not done with a sense of responsibility and humanity. My primary focus in this book, though, is on the here and now and on *how* the most powerful mental health enterprise in the world—the American Psychiatric Association—is defining *abnormality, mental illness*, or *mental disorder*, rather than on the definitions' consequences. The point is not that decisions about who is normal are riddled with personal biases and political considerations but rather that, by dint of a handful of influential professionals' efforts, those subjective determinants of diagnoses masquerade as solid science and truth.

There is a great deal that is or can be good in psychotherapy, and some people, for whatever reasons, feel more comfortable turning to a therapist than to friends or family for help with certain kinds of problems. Whether with a social worker, psychiatrist, psychiatric nurse, counselor, or psychologist, if the person seeking help and the person designated as a helper happen to "click" interpersonally and emotionally, if the latter truly cares about the former and thinks conscientiously about what is happening in the therapy sessions, the process can be fascinating and positive, and the outcome can be quite wonderful. Many fine books and papers have been written about how to conduct psychotherapy with compassion and intelligence, and I refer interested readers to them. But that is not the subject of this book. I would ask readers to do me the favor of remembering, as you read my book, that this is neither an antipsychiatry nor a "Let's-trash-all-therapists" book. Its main focus is quite specifically on the disingenuous and dishonest process of constructing the world's most influential handbook of "mental disorders."

This book is also not much about whether most of what is called mental illness has a biological basis or about the "medicalization" of what Thomas Szasz refers to as people's "problems in living," although I do refer to this issue several times. I *do* believe that there may be some biological or physiological basis for some of the things that are currently called psychiatric disorders. However, so much of the research on these possible causes is so deeply flawed that it seems dangerous to draw very definite conclusions about them. R. Walter Heinrichs, for instance, recently wrote a thoughtful review of seventy years of research on what "schizophrenia" might be, how variously "it" has been defined, what might cause "it," and what "treatments" might be helpful for "it." His conclusion was that very little is known or understood and that the label still suffers from what he calls "a heterogeneity problem," a polite way of saying it is so variously applied that it is losing much of its meaning. This is particularly worrying both because research in this area has such a long history and because it has generally been assumed that whatever "schizophrenia" is, it is known to be genetically based. Now, it appears, what seemed certain is not.

When responsible reviews of research about diagnosis and treatment of mental disorders are carefully conducted, uncertainty is often the result. Much of what is labeled "mental illness" would more appropriately be called problems in living, and some has been shown to result from such problems as dietary deficiencies or from food or environmental allergies. What *is* important for this book is that, although some *DSM* diagnoses supposedly have some physical origin (hormonal, genetic, brain-based, etc.) and others supposedly result from people's experiences in their families or their allegedly "sick" kinds of motives and feelings, *all* of that labeling is based on the *DSM* folks' choices about whom to declare abnormal. As psychologist Carol Tavris has observed, "the DSM is not called the 'Diagnostic and Statistical Manual of Mental Disorders and a

Whole Bunch of Everyday Problems in Living.'" It is marketed simply as a manual of mental disorders.

I do not claim that everyday problems are the only reasons that people might display what are classified as the symptoms of mental illness, and I do not claim to understand all of the possible sources of such troubles. However, I do believe that some of the masses of money, time, and energy spent in developing, revising, and marketing the *DSM* might be more productively used in exploring other possible causes of people's troubles. Furthermore, much of the time and energy that professionals who use the *DSM* invest in learning about and trying to apply its contents could be more usefully invested in such endeavors as paying careful, caring attention to what one's patients say and working, free from dogma, to understand what helps them. (In the *DSM*, the authors do not even address the question of what treatments might help with which kinds of problems.) But today, in most settings where new generations of psychiatrists and other physicians, social workers, psychologists, and psychiatric nurses are trained, the *DSM* is *the* key volume about mental illness that all trainees must learn from cover to cover. It is also used as *the* key volume for a great deal of the research on mental health and mental illnesses funded by government agencies and private foundations. For years, I had—somewhat tongue-in-cheek—described the *DSM* as the "bible of mental health professionals." Then I saw an advertisement in which a book about the *DSM* was promoted with this quotation from Donald Godwin, chairman and professor in the Department of Psychiatry at the University of Kansas: "Like all semireligious works, DSM-III needs an exegesis."

When mental health authorities are asked questions on television and radio phone-in shows, they often refer to the *DSM* as though it were scientifically proven gospel, as though saying "It is here in the *DSM*" makes it true. The *DSM* is a weighty volume in both its sheer physical size (nearly three pounds) and the aura of scientific precision that emanates from it: Each diagnostic category has a multidigit number attached to it, a list of criteria, and a "cutoff point" indicating that in order to warrant this particular label, a person must meet, for instance, six of the nine criteria listed. In any debate in Western culture, it usually strengthens one's position to claim that one is scientific, rational, and objective, while the other side is "politically motivated," irrational, and subjective. Although increasing numbers of people recognize that complete objectivity is impossible and that even seemingly rational claims that scientists make about their research are often both politically and emotionally motivated, the tendency to accept high-status medical scientists' and practitioners' words as truth is still widespread. Nearly always, those who have the most power—such as the APA—are those who claim to be objective and have the easiest time persuading people to accept that claim.

The *DSM* is also big business for its publisher, the APA: A recent revision yielded more than a million dollars in revenue, since each time a new edition appears, libraries and many practicing therapists—both psychiatrists and others—and mental health researchers have to buy the updated version. The 1987 edition was translated into Chinese, Danish, Dutch, Finnish, French, German, Greek, Hungarian, Italian, Japanese, Norwegian, Portuguese, Russian, Spanish, Swedish, Turkish, and Ukrainian. Related products are also marketed, including "various casebooks, tape cassettes, minimanuals, workshops, interview protocols, and computer programs." Products marketed for the previous edition and the current one include casebooks, interview guides, a study guide, a sourcebook, an audiotape, a videotape, a training guide, and several computer software packages.

Insurance companies, general practitioners, and lawyers make frequent use of the manual, insurance companies to decide which patients to reimburse for their inpatient or outpatient treatments. In fact, it has been described as "a surprising runaway best-seller, primarily because of sales to nonpsychiatrists," whose numbers are legion. Kirk and Kutchins report that between 1975 and 1990,

> the number of psychiatrists increased from 26 to 36 thousand, clinical psychologists from 15 to 42 thousand, clinical social workers from 25 to 80 thousand, and marriage and family counselors from 6 to 40 thousand. In aggregate, the increase in 15 years has been from 72 to 198 thousand professionals in just those four professions (Goleman, 1990). Similarly, in NIMH-surveyed psychiatric facilities, the number of personnel increased from 375 thousand in 1976 to 441 thousand by 1984 (Schulberg & Manderscheid, 1989, p. 16).

In all, the *DSM-III-R* is reported to have sold about 1.1 million copies in less than six years.

Although my focus is on the *DSM*, I could not attempt in a single book to address the vast array of its biases, examples of sloppiness and illogical thinking, and just plain silliness. I do hope that readers who wish to learn about more than I have covered here will have a look at some of the excellent books and papers on this subject listed in the bibliography.

As I have written elsewhere, I believe that far too many people who are badly treated because of their race, sex, age, class, sexual orientation, mental or physical condition, physical appearance, and so on end up seeking psychotherapy because they mistakenly believe that their unhappiness stems from something within themselves. Too much contemporary treatment by mental health professionals, including treatment influenced by the *DSM*, maintains this almost exclusive focus on individuals' psyches, as if the major sources of their troubles came from within them.

I do not intend for this book to destroy anyone or any institution. Rather, I long for it to help reveal the truth and encourage the openness and honesty of the individuals and institutions that represent themselves to the public as members of the helping professions who will assist them with their troubles. Without complete honesty and openness and without high moral and scientific standards and an overriding emphasis on understanding how we affect the people we purport to help, we cannot truly help, and they ought not to trust us when we say that we shall. As Jerome Frank has written, "The unattainability of the ideal is no excuse for shirking the effort to obtain the best available."

Certainly, some people hurt themselves or hurt or frighten others. Some people suffer intense emotional pain, some are outcasts, some are out of touch with what most people would consider reality. All of this is terribly sad and worrying, and as a society, we must find ways to alleviate these problems. I do not claim to know how best to do so. I honestly don't know, when I see someone screaming that thousands of bugs are crawling over him or that she is getting special messages from St. Jude, why that is happening. I certainly don't claim to know how to take away the anguish and confusion of everyone who feels them, and this book is not about that. But it does relate to all of these people, kinds of problems, and feelings, and how they are dealt with. And I do know that *DSM*-type enterprises have not been much help in alleviating human suffering. As a specialist in research methods, I want people to know how sparse are the research and even the logical thinking on which this diagnostic manual is based. I also want it known that researchers have found very few answers to these questions through using labels of mental illness.

I do intend this to be an anti-elitism book, since I want us all to be able to make an informed assessment of the people we allow to decide whether or not you and I and our loved ones are normal. Rarely are mental health professionals questioned about how they decide which people and what behavior are normal, and too rarely do the professionals themselves think critically about what they do. Laypeople generally hesitate to question those who seem to be experts in a mystifying or highly technical field; to do such questioning can feel like asking the clergy if there really is a God. It can also feel presumptuous: "Who am I to question someone who went to school for so many years and learned about all of this stuff? My questions will probably be stupid. And what if my questioning just makes the person angry?" Reluctance to question authorities tends to intensify when, as with mental health professionals, we see them in a time of desperate need. As I have written elsewhere, there is a whole panoply of reasons that the therapists and researchers themselves so often fail to think critically and questioningly about what they do. Questions that are rarely asked come to seem unworthy of being asked, unjustified, or unwarranted, and so the question of who is normal and who can legitimately answer that question is seldom raised. I hope that this book will encourage readers to overcome this kind of reluctance to question. We need not hesitate to think critically about what therapists and therapy researchers say and do, because, as Carol Mithers has noted, "Although the discipline presents itself as a 'science,' its entire history is one of a series of new techniques and schools of thought." Therapy has been defined as an "unidentified technique applied to unspecified problems with unpredictable outcomes," and longtime psychotherapy researcher Hans Strupp has written: "Psychotherapy has become a billion-dollar industry . . . lacking clear boundaries, with hazy quality control and relatively vague ethical standards."

Identifying herself as a former mental patient, Judi Chamberlin has written: "Leaving the determination of whether mental illness exists strictly to the psychiatrists is like leaving the determination of the validity of astrology in the hands of professional astrologers. While occasional psychiatrists (or astrologers) may question the very basis of the discipline they practice, such behavior is understandably rare, since people are unlikely to question the underlying premises of their occupations, in which they often have a large financial and emotional stake."

Before we look at what the *DSM* group did, I think I ought to describe my attitude toward authorities and experts. Through almost all of the years of my formal education, from nursery school until partway through graduate school, I assumed that authorities knew best and held dearly the interests of those over whom they had power. I believed this so fervently (and sometimes obnoxiously, I suspect) that I was the kind of child who thought students who threw spitballs when the teacher briefly left the classroom were lacking in moral fiber. Rare experiences in high school, occasional ones in college, and most of my graduate school experiences revealed to me that authorities' motives are not always altruistic and their procedures not always fair or logical. By now, more than two decades after finishing graduate school, my work increasingly involves questioning authorities and experts, but I find that I nevertheless tend, like most people, to start by assuming that those who have power are right—and that they do the right thing. I realize that this may sound strange, coming from someone who has been called antiauthoritarian and radically feminist, but each time I find that an authority has behaved irresponsibly or has lied or has been cruel, I feel a renewed sense of disappointment. I wish the world were a safer place than it is. It gave me no pleasure, then, to watch the unfolding of the disturbing story of how the *DSM* authors decide who is normal, but I tell it here because I do believe that the truth helps make us free.

They Say You're Crazy

1
How *Do* They Decide Who Is Normal?

Labels assigned by medical professionals can consign individuals to the scorn of others, and to the physical and emotional abuse that may follow.
—Martha Minow, "Interpreting Rights"

Only in psychiatry is the existence of physical disease determined by APA presidential proclamations, by committee decisions, and even, at times, by a vote of the members of APA, not to mention the courts.
—Peter Breggin, *Toxic Psychiatry*

If we allow others to decide whether or not we are normal, we lose the power to define, to judge, and, often, to respect ourselves. Today in North America, classifying people as normal or abnormal is a major enterprise that is carried out on many levels, from the American Psychiatric Association (APA) to school personnel to next-door neighbors. So many people fear and worry in silence about whether they are normal that there is no way to assess the devastation caused and the energy drained by these concerns.

Jumping up and down with excitement, five-year-old Tommy says, "Guess what, Daddy? I got to help Mommy make the roast!" His father's answering silence, the way his jaw muscles tense on one side and the light leaves his eyes, ensure that this child will not want to cook again. Tommy may not understand for many years that the switch from delight to discomfort that he felt came from his father's feelings about what a normal boy should and should not do.

Whenever nine-year-old Julia notices other girls her age looking at her, she thinks it means that something is wrong with her, that she is not normal.

In his first year of junior high school, Benjamin learned for the first time that, in writing an essay, it is neither usual nor necessary to have every word in mind before putting pen to paper. Until then, he had felt intense anxiety as he tried to work the way he thought most people worked, the correct way, the normal way.

At puberty, Marilyn was ashamed about the blue veins in her growing breasts and Stan was ashamed of the blue veins in his growing penis. Marilyn had never seen other women's breasts up close, and Stan had never looked carefully at other men's penises. Both assumed that their bodies were different from everyone else's, that they were not normal.

After Esther and Robert fell in love and began living together, their first major fight was over towels. In the home where Esther grew up, everyone used a fresh towel for each shower, but in Robert's home towels were changed weekly. Esther believed it was a filthy habit not to change towels often, and Robert believed it was wasteful to do so. Until they discussed their feelings of amazement when they discovered each other's different beliefs, each one simply thought that the other's attitude was abnormal.

About once a month, Penny feels that she is terribly and unjustifiably irritable. Two doctors have told her that she has premenstrual syndrome and that most women do. She has wrestled with the question, "If I'm so irritable, does that mean I'm not normal?" and then with the question, "But if most women get this way, are most women abnormal?" and then, "Are women who do not *get this way normal or abnormal?" "What is a normal woman?" "Does being a woman mean being abnormal?"*

When Harold finds the cutthroat atmosphere at work distasteful, he fears that his reaction means that he is not a real man, that he is not normal. He wonders, "If acting like a man makes me unhappy, can I *be a man and be happy?"*

In spite of the women's movement, when Ramona's first child is born and, during six weeks of maternity leave, she feels sometimes scared, sometimes bored, sometimes desperate, and always exhausted, she fears that she is not a real woman, that she is not normal.

Eleanor was beaten repeatedly by her husband and became depressed as a result. She sought therapy because of the depression, and her therapist "taught" her that she was undoubtedly provoking her husband to beat her, since she unconsciously "needed" to suffer. She had never enjoyed the beatings, but when she told her therapist that, he replied that her enjoyment was unconscious: It was there but she just wasn't aware of it. Eleanor had always been told that a good woman stands by her man and tames his rages if necessary, but she had been unable to help her husband learn to control his anger, so she felt like a failure as a woman, an abnormal one. Hearing then from a respected authority that she unconsciously enjoyed suffering, she had further reason to feel psychologically twisted. "How grotesque I am," she thought, "to enjoy suffering. I must be terri-

bly abnormal." Her husband does not wonder very much about whether it is normal for him to be abusive, nor does she.

When Don is feeling about as stressed as most of us frequently feel, he believes this is evidence that, like his father before him, he will have a psychotic break and commit suicide. At times when many people would think to themselves, "I am under so much pressure. I need to go for a run or take the weekend and relax," Don instantly interprets such feelings as signals that he is dangerously abnormal.

A woman with great artistic talents and sensibilities felt a sense of panic because she had become extremely angry at her boyfriend and had envisioned blood dripping down in the air in front of her. She panicked because she labeled that image a hallucination and concluded that she was possibly going crazy or, at the very least, was certainly not normal.

When I was a psychotherapist, I found that, in one way or another, I spent an enormous amount of time urging people to stop worrying about whether or not they were normal. Graham Berman, a deeply caring psychiatrist, has observed, "Often, when I make a *descriptive* remark, the patient responds as though it had been *evaluative*." His comment hit home for me, as both therapist and layperson. As a therapist, how often have I said something like, "Since you feel things very deeply—" and before I could say another word, the patient has burst out, "Yes, I *know* I am too intense!" Or, many people would tell me, "I know it's not normal for me to be missing my husband so much. After all, it's been a whole year since he died." Many times I have spoken with people whose experiences caused them anguish, fear, or sadness and who were burdened unnecessarily with the idea that their feelings were excessive or even wrong. As a result, their time and energy were drained by their attempts to force their feelings to fit a mold that they believed to be normal.

I myself have not escaped such worries without a great deal of effort, for in our culture there are so many unwritten rules about which kinds (and what quantities) of feelings and behavior are normal. To make matters worse, on a continuum of expressive-to-inexpressive societies, North America's Western European–influenced culture sits far toward the emotionally controlled, inexpressive end. Of course, not all judgments about psychological normality—whether by therapists or by other people—are based on the degree of expressiveness. Other standards of normality have to do with the degree to which the person is regarded as "in touch with reality" (however variously *reality* may be defined), the clarity of the person's thinking (in the eyes of the person making the judgment), and so on.

Where do we get our ideas of which people and what behavior are normal? There is an unfortunately large number of such sources, from parents' tense and silent disapproval all the way to official declarations in the allegedly scientifically based tome of diagnoses, the *Diagnostic and Statistical Manual of Mental Disorders* (*DSM*). Other sources include the media, religion, information from friends or books—or *lack* of information or misinformation—about other people's experiences, limitations (for many reasons) in our knowledge about various possibilities for feeling and behaving, and (for various possible reasons) a narrow view of what is normal. Then, too, it sometimes seems as though everyone is either a therapist, a therapy patient, or both.

We cannot help but be affected by our loved ones', teachers', or employers' beliefs about whether or not we are normal. The degree to which we are affected depends on such factors as how much power they have over us, how much we care about them, how much we respect their opinions, how normal we consider them to be, and how insecure we are. What does it say about "normality" when we read an official announcement that "the government" sent out a team of researchers in the United States that found "that nearly half of all Americans experience a psychiatric disorder at least once in their lifetime," 14 percent have three or more, and 30 percent have had one in the preceding year alone? (And this study was based on only *some* of the many disorders included in the *DSM*.) Millions of people are called abnormal in a government-funded study, and countless others fear or believe that they, too, are abnormal. If only half of us have no (diagnosed) psychiatric disorder, then does that mean no one is normal, since in one everyday sense *normal* means "like most people"? Do these statistics take the meaning right out of *normality*? If fully half of "them" are abnormal, how can we not be scared that we, too, might secretly fit that description? Or does it mean that we live in such a crazy-making, sick, impersonal society that it does serious psychological damage to half of us? And if the latter is the case, should we be calling that "disordered" 50 percent "mentally ill," as though the problem arose from and resides within them, or should we instead call them society's wounded?

Since entering graduate school in clinical psychology in 1969, when all sorts of assumptions about the way authorities were running the world were being questioned, I have been fascinated by how people decide who is normal. As a first-year graduate student, I taught an undergraduate honors seminar on concepts of normality. Nearly ten years later, when asked to teach a women's studies course about how psychologists study sex and gender issues, I began my lectures by discussing psychologists' assumptions about what were normal attitudes, emotions, and abilities for females and how those assumptions differed from those about males.

In 1984 I wrote an article called "The Myth of Women's Masochism," in which I argued that the common claim that normal women enjoy suffering was both unfounded and seriously damaging to women. In 1985, while I was waiting for my book of the same name to be published, this work drew me into the heart of a powerful institution's debates about who is normal. I received a phone call from psychiatrist Jean Baker Miller, who informed me that the influential American Psychiatric Association had decided to create a category of psychiatric abnormality called "Masochistic Personality Disorder" (MPD). I was both stunned and appalled, and from that moment I began opposing their official adoption of that category. My opposition was based partly on the absence of undistorted evidence that people enjoy suffering—in contrast to feeling that some suffering or endurance is necessary to get what they actually do enjoy, such as working for a paycheck or acquiescing to a husband's unreasonable demands in order to keep peace in the family. I was also concerned because the concept of masochism had been used for a long time, most often to distort women's motives and behavior so that they seemed bizarre and sick. Frequently, a woman who stayed with a battering husband was assumed to enjoy the pain, and a woman rape victim was assumed to have brought the rape on herself. Few women who were suffering or unhappy escaped being pathologized, treated as abnormal, in this way; women who denied that they wanted to be hurt were said to be *unconscious* masochists. The legacy of Sigmund Freud and his disciples, who asserted that masochism was an essential, normal characteristic of women, remained strong. Another

serious concern about the APA's new category was that
many women who had been raised to be traditional "good
wives" were going to have that behavior stamped as abnormal, because putting other people's needs ahead of one's
own without being appreciated was part of the MPD
description.

While opposing the APA's move to include Masochistic
Personality Disorder in their diagnostic handbook, I
learned that they also planned to classify many women as
premenstrually psychiatrically ill, under the label "Premenstrual Dysphoric Disorder." In spite of massive protests, the APA went ahead and included both categories
in the 1987 edition of their heavy, impressive-looking diagnostic manual, the *Diagnostic and Statistical Manual of
Mental Disorders III-R* (*DSM-III-R*: third edition, revised).
After that time, I continued to work with others to urge
the APA to exclude the categories from the 1994 edition,
the *DSM-IV*. Between the two editions, I was asked to
advise the *DSM-IV* committees on MPD (under a new
label) and the premenstrual category, as they reviewed the
research and decided whether to continue to declare that
these two kinds of abnormality were real. As a result of
that work, I got an inside look at how this august body
decides who is normal, and what I saw disturbed me
deeply. I was shocked to realize how little I, as a mental
health professional, had known about how authorities in
my own field went about choosing whom to classify as
mentally ill. I realized that, despite my early interest in
the idea of normality, I had hardly questioned the way
certain behavior comes to be called normal or abnormal.
And the more I have seen of the devastating consequences
of being considered abnormal, the more concerned I have
become. Some therapists claim that "mental disorder" is
not necessarily the same as "abnormality," but in fact to

most therapists and most laypeople, the terms "mental disorder," "mental illness," and "mental or emotional abnormality" are interchangeable.

What Happens When We Think We Are Not Normal?

Being labeled abnormal has determined how countless people feel about themselves. Some people have been deeply scarred because of the labeling itself, as well as by harmful "treatments" that result. Many people feel needless shame, fear, panic, conflict, and anger when messages that they are not normal are conveyed either formally or informally—by an official diagnosis, a comment from a family member, or the rolling eyes of others in meetings or classes in response to their remarks. The labeling also has far-reaching consequences in terms of practical and formal decisions about those classified as abnormal, and those decisions in turn can have devastating emotional as well as practical results. Labels figure prominently in decisions about whose psychotherapy will be paid for by their insurance companies, who will be hospitalized against their will, who may be declared by a court of law to be incompetent or too disturbed to have custody of their children, who will be allowed to grant or withhold permission to perform surgery on their bodies, and on and on and on.

A cavalier unconcern about such consequences is too often the response of powerful mental health professionals who create categories of abnormality. In a recent public debate, spokespeople for the American Psychiatric Association were asked why they intended to declare premenstrual syndrome a psychiatric disorder, when their own committee of PMS experts had concluded that the research on the subject had been poorly done and the sparse data were only "preliminary." They were requested to respond to the public's expression of alarm about the harm done to women by such labeling and were given examples of women with whom I had spoken or who had sent letters to me, whose serious, painful pelvic infections had gone undiagnosed and untreated while doctors said they were simply premenstrually mentally ill; who had become depressed and attempted suicide due to antidepressants given to them by doctors when they reported having PMS; and who stayed with abusive husbands because the men threatened, "If you leave me, I'll get custody of the kids, because everyone knows you're sick in the head with PMS."

Incredibly, after hearing such reports, the top APA officials and leaders of the diagnostic handbook committee claimed they had found no evidence that any woman had been harmed by being called premenstrually psychiatrically disordered. Technically, perhaps, that was correct: *They* had found no such evidence themselves, perhaps because they had not sought it; their lengthy report on PMS research includes no mention of any attempt to find out whether women had been harmed by being assigned this kind of diagnosis. But even after they were told about women who had been harmed, they continued to deny publicly that any harm had been done (see Chapter 5). Trying to give the impression that the only harm done was from the public's stigmatizing of people called mentally ill, they would discuss no other kinds of harm and instead preached that stigmatizing is wrong. In this way, the world's most influential psychiatric organization irresponsibly said simply that there *ought* to be no negative fallout from their actions and then ignored evidence of such fallout, without taking responsible steps to ensure that no one else would be unjustifiably categorized as abnormal. It was like making someone wear a sign saying "I have an infectious disease" and then self-righteously standing aside, proclaiming that no one should shun the allegedly diseased individual. It reflected a profound lack of understanding of (or, perhaps, concern about) how it feels and how it affects one to be labeled abnormal. The architects of the *DSM* do not say that they aim to stamp people with pejorative images, and some of them seem disconcerted by the news that this is a frequent consequence of their work; but its frequency is undeniable, and people in the "helping professions" surely ought to take some responsibility for minimizing, rather than denying, the negative results of their actions.

When terms like *abnormal* or *mentally ill* are spoken, what kinds of images come to mind? Usually, images of difference and alienation, suggesting that "they" are not as competent, human, or safe to be around as the rest of "us." And often, "abnormal" and "mentally ill" are equated with "crazy," a label that calls forth images of someone who is out of control, out of touch with "reality," incapable of forming a good relationship, untrustworthy, quite possibly dangerous, and probably not worth one's attention, time, or energy.

If such labeling had some positive effects, it might be worth risking the negative consequences for those who are labeled abnormal. The professionals most concerned with labeling claim that they assign people to categories of mental illness so that they will know how to help them. If such assignment to categories really did help very much, that would indeed be encouraging, but treatment of emotional problems and conflicts is very different from medical or surgical treatment. If I broke a limb, I would want to be properly diagnosed as having a broken arm so that the surgeon would not mistakenly set and put a cast on my leg. But diagnosing individuals as mentally ill has not been shown to do much to alleviate their anguish and indeed often makes it worse. It is not wrong to recognize when people need help, but sorting them into categories of normal vs. abnormal is not necessary and, at this stage, rarely helpful.

How It Feels to Be Told We Are Normal

When I was a therapist, I continually heard from patients that the most important moments in our work together had been the times when I had assured them that they were not crazy, not even unusual in the ways that they were feeling or acting. A woman who had been a long-term patient on a psychiatric ward in the Midwest told me recently that no therapist or other mental health worker ever told her that she was normal. For her, the important moment came when "something inside myself told me, after years of damaging drug treatments, that I did not need fixing because I was not broken. And that was the moment when I began to feel better and take control of my life."

In keeping with this approach, I have always tried to avoid using the word "normal," even to reassure people who sought my help that they were fine, because I thought that might encourage them to focus on the whole question of "Am I normal or abnormal?" Instead, I was more likely to say that what they were feeling or doing seemed perfectly understandable to me in view of what had happened, that I knew many people who had felt or behaved in similar ways, or sometimes that I had, too. One woman described how coldly her husband had treated her and then hastened to explain, "He really doesn't *mean* to hurt me. It's just that he had a terrible childhood." She had been trying so hard to be a loving, patient wife that she had ignored her feelings of rejection, hurt, and, ultimately, anger at him. She was quite certain that those were not feelings a "normal, unselfish" woman would have, in view of all that her husband had suffered forty years before. When I told her that I found her feelings completely understandable, she was able to stop worrying about whether or not she was normal and to start thinking about her own needs. She told me that she also felt intense relief at being able to save the energy she had been putting into wrestling with the question of whether she was abnormally self-centered and impatient and instead to invest that energy in thinking about what might work for her and possibly for their relationship.

I firmly believe that what is called "psychotherapy" might be more helpful more often if "being in therapy" were not associated in so many people's minds with being abnormal, deficient, or defective. Because those associations are so strong, many therapy patients listen to their therapists' remarks or suggestions and interpret them not simply as interesting perspectives or useful advice but also as signs that they themselves are so damaged that they have to have such help.

Having a therapist help take your focus off questions related to whether or not you are normal can be liberating and energizing. When I was in therapy many years ago, I was going through a divorce and taking care of my two children while also working at a full-time, paid job. I often felt overwhelmed by and inadequate to the tasks I was trying to carry out. Fortunately, my caring therapist allowed me to phone him at home when I felt the need to do so. Several times within a month, I called him at home when I was feeling especially desperate. Back in his office during a scheduled appointment, I told him I felt ashamed for having phoned him. "Each time I called you, I felt fine as soon as I heard your voice," I said, "and I know that means I am just terribly dependent." He replied calmly—

and, I realized, accurately—"I don't believe it means that you are dependent. I think that you have come to associate me with certain strengths in yourself, and you were calling me to remind yourself of those strengths." What a beautiful gift was that reply. I felt better about myself, my shame evaporated, and I was energized.

In a similar vein, after I wrote *The Myth of Women's Masochism*, a woman called to say, "I had been in therapy for eight years, and every week, after I told him how unhappy I was feeling, my therapist would nod wisely and say, 'Do you see how you bring your misery on yourself?' . . . I had become more and more depressed and more and more certain that I had no one to blame but myself. Then, one day, I turned on the radio partway through a program [and] the first words I heard were, '. . . and I have never met a woman who actually liked to suffer.' At the sound of your words, I felt a weight lift from my shoulders for the first time in all those years. I quit therapy and . . . *knew* I could change my life for the better, because some stranger on the radio had said she didn't believe I enjoyed suffering."

Marilyn and Stan, who worried about the blue veins on their developing bodies, both found out from friends that there was nothing unusual about their body parts. As a result, they felt far less grotesque and frightened. In fact, some important cross-cultural research suggests that when people's distress is labeled in ways that encourage their return to better functioning rather than categorize them as having long-lasting abnormalities, they feel better sooner.[7]

Because believing oneself to be abnormal can be so damaging, it is crucial to be aware of how we come to judge ourselves and others as normal and abnormal. In this book, I shall concentrate primarily on the APA, the Western world's most powerful organization that makes these judgments in a formal, official way. I chose that focus both because so much power is concentrated in their hands and because knowing how they work can help us understand the bases and assumptions involved in less formal labeling, such as by our family members, friends, and coworkers.

First, I shall describe the extent of power and influence of the APA's handbook of "mental disorder," the *DSM*. Then, in Chapter 2, I describe some of the ways one might, in principle, decide who is normal. In Chapter 3 I address the question "Does the mental health establishment believe *anyone* is normal?" In Chapters 4, 5, and 6 I tell the disturbing story of how the APA has actually made irresponsible decisions about who is normal in some recent cases. Chapter 7 is about the false aura of scientific precision that surrounds the *DSM*—where it comes from and why it is misleading—and Chapter 8 is my attempt to explain *why* mental health experts take such a slapdash approach to classifying people as abnormal. In Chapter 9 I describe the way the media help support the *DSM*, and in Chapter 10 I make some concluding remarks.

First, let us look at why the *DSM* warrants special attention.

The Ideal and the Actual: Why Focus on the *DSM*?

It was through the development of a new psychiatric manual that research psychiatrists, by emphasizing the sorry state of diagnostic reliability and its significance and, further, by claiming that they could do better, positioned themselves near the center of American psychiatry.

—Stuart Kirk and Herb Kutchins, *The Selling of DSM*

Matching Treatment to Problem

I won't recount here the histories of the professions that assign psychological or psychiatric diagnoses—social workers, psychiatric nurses, counselors of various kinds, psychologists, psychiatrists, and so on. I want instead to look at where we are now, what happens now with the process of diagnosis. When people go to or are brought to a mental health professional, it is because they want to change their feelings or behavior or because someone else wants them to do so. It is widely assumed that once a therapist knows what a patient's problems are, it will be obvious what kind of treatment will help. However, that is not the case. If all therapists told their prospective patients, "People come to me with all sorts of problems, and I have been able to help only some kinds of people with only certain kinds of problems, and I will be glad to *try* to help you," that would be all right, but many therapists do nothing of the kind. It would especially be all right if therapists either said, "Frankly, I am judging how much I have been able to help people in a very subjective and haphazard way, on the basis of how they tell me they feel, how I think they have changed, and what I hear from some of them, occasionally, years after they stop seeing me" or if they said, "Carefully done scientific research has shown that if I do X with you, the result will be Y." However, few therapists volunteer the first kind of information (accurate though it is for most therapists), and the latter is usually not true. Masses of research have been done by and about mental health professionals and the work we do, but very little has been well done, and even less has produced conclusive or even very reliable information. And too often, treatments are not based on the better research. For instance, a recent study of patients in psychiatric hospitals showed minimal relationships among the way a patient was diagnosed, the patient's problems, and the kinds of drugs that were prescribed. This finding was particularly important in light of the fact that psychotropic drugs were the primary form of treatment. That drugs were the primary treatment is all the more alarming because many of those patients' problems are not of the kinds usually thought of as psychiatric symptoms.

In private practice, therapists may be more thoughtful and responsible about suiting the treatment to the problem, or they may not be, and when they are not, because they work alone they are less subject to the scrutiny of colleagues or nurses who in hospital settings might possibly question their approaches. This is not to say that all therapists are incompetent and irresponsible but simply that the frequency of incompetency and irresponsibility constitutes a very different picture from the general public's assumption that therapists know what they are doing and that they base their treatment on absolute, scientifically proven truths. In fact, most of the effective work in the mental health system is based on the strengths of the therapist-patient relationship and on the judgments, feelings, and intuitions of each party. Occasionally, some people may be helped by some drugs, but what is most relevant to the issue at hand is that very little is known about which drugs might help whom and under what circumstances. I don't question honest, well-executed attempts to find some certainty or guidelines for helping people feel better. But so much of the *DSM* enterprise has nothing to do with that.

Nine years ago, I had my own experience with a treatment that not only did not help me but actually hurt me. I had learned that a dear friend was dying and was so upset that I was having trouble sleeping. Coincidentally, it turned out, I was having some breathing problems. A friend urged me to see a doctor about the breathing problems, and I did. Although I learned much later that they were simply part of an allergic reaction, the doctor asked me what else was going on in my life, and when I told him, he wanted to prescribe a drug for me. "I won't take Valium, and I don't like drugs in general," I told him, but he replied, "I'm not giving you Valium, just a little something that has no side effects at all. It will help you sleep. If you continue to lose sleep, that will just make everything worse." When I continued to demur, he promised to prescribe only five pills, one for each of the next five nights. There I was, an experienced psychologist who had never taken medication for an emotional upset and did not want to, and I didn't think that that was what I was doing. He had said this was just to help me sleep. The day after I took the first pill, I went from being terribly sad about my friend's illness to finding myself with tears streaming down my cheeks without warning, intermittently, all day long. Fortunately, just by chance, I had an appointment the next day with my naturopath and told her what was happening. She asked for the name of the medication, I told her it was called Halcion, and she checked and found out that depression is one of its common effects. I immediately stopped taking the Halcion, and the tearfulness ceased. The physician had meant well, I am sure, but he was not thinking carefully enough—or not checking the drug's side effects carefully enough—to realize that giving a person who is feeling sad a drug that can cause depression ought to be considered a certifiably insane act!

I tell this story because, once a person's emotional upsets are classified as psychiatric, the chances that psychiatric treatments will be recommended skyrocket. And psychiatric treatments consist these days primarily of drugs, psychotherapy, and shock treatments. The first and last have well-documented risks and dangers for most people, and psychotherapy is not always conducted thoughtfully, intelligently, or humanely. Again, I would not deny anyone the chance to seek therapy or try other treatments, but it is time for consumers to know that the likelihood of finding helpful and not harmful treatment through traditional mental health professionals is not as great as we tend to believe and that diagnostic classification has not helped very much.

As a former and now occasional therapist, I can say that when my patients feel better, if I am honest with myself, I often cannot be sure why. It is virtually impossible to do good research on what works in psychotherapy, because once you intervene in order to study therapy, you have already changed it, so you don't know what to make of the results. When I have worked on mental health teams, I have observed repeatedly that the conclusions about causes of patients' problems and recommendations for treatment depended a great deal on which team members had official power and authority or who had the guts to speak up. When we add to the uncertainty about helpful treatments the closely guarded secret that patients often do not get better, we realize how crucial it is to think carefully about why the major diagnostic handbook is assumed to contain the truth.

There are questions that must be asked, moral and political questions, but also practical questions about what we are doing when we enter the diagnostic arena.

First, what are the kinds of reasons one would want to change oneself or want someone else to change, and are some of those reasons more morally desirable than others? For instance, am I on higher moral ground if I want to overcome my shyness in order to be able to reach out to others and help them or if I want to overcome my shyness in order to feel less frightened when I walk into a cocktail party? Am I on higher moral ground if I suggest that a friend take her son to a therapist so he can figure out how to deal with his father's death or if I suggest that a friend take her son to a therapist so the therapist will teach him to sit still at the dinner table? What goals are worthy uses of a therapist's and a patient's time? What goals are likely to increase the patient's options, freedom, and comfort, and what goals are likely to limit them? Should a therapist always agree to try to help make change happen when a patient seeks, or is brought for, assistance in doing that? Should I try to help someone stop feeling guilty for having copied one answer on a sixth-grade science test ten years before? Should I help that man stop feeling guilty for having left his wife when he learned she had breast cancer? What about helping a man stop feeling guilty for having told his wife he really wished she would agree to have another child, just when she was preparing to begin her college career? Psychiatrist Peter Breggin has written, "Psychiatry is the institution socially mandated to respond to personal helplessness and failure." Fair enough, but do we want to equate personal helplessness and failure with mental disorder? And should the province of therapists be only "mental disorder," or should it also include "problems in living," however one defines both of those terms?

Second, can the professionals whom people ask for help in changing actually provide that help? In principle, this question could be answered by careful scientific research. All kinds of therapists using a whole range of therapy techniques with the whole possible range of patients could be studied, so that we could find out which kinds of therapists could help which kinds of people with which problems and how that could best be done. But such research would require staggering amounts of money and very long periods of time. Some researchers have tried to do some corners of this major project, but rarely have their studies been well done. And when studies are not well done, it is impossible to know whether their results reveal some important information or whether they should be taken with many grains of salt.

Ideally, we would accurately and carefully list the problems and personality characteristics of everyone who seeks the help of mental health professionals. Then, we would study masses of these people in terms of which treatments and which kinds of therapists helped them, pour all the information into a computer, subject it to sophisticated statistical analyses, and find out at the end that if you, being the kind of person and therapist you are, see X kind of patient with Y kind of problem, and use treatment Z, there is an 80 percent chance you will be able to help. But as we shall see in the course of this book, we are light-years from being able to do that. Humans' psychological functioning is so complex and unpredictable that current scientific techniques can reveal only a fraction of what therapists need to know. There has been little well-done scientific research about what helps, and what has been done is often inaccurately reported because it is presented by drug companies or groups that have various stakes in the research. None of that would matter if some of our colleagues, associations, and institutions did not work so hard to give the impression that more is known than really is.

Because science has not yet given us the answer, moral questions then arise:

- Do some (or many) therapists intentionally or unintentionally deceive themselves and their patients about their ability to help?
- How do therapists decide whether or not to agree

to work on the goals set by the patient (or the person who wants the patient to have therapy)?

- Do therapists think carefully about the research that has been done in regard to what is helpful to whom? Do they use that in making decisions about their clinical work?
- Whether or not they refer to the relevant research, do therapists take the trouble to follow up on their patients' progress once the therapy has ended? (Few therapists do.) If not, they cannot be sure whether what they have done has been helpful, harmful, or ineffectual.

And most important:

- Which therapists are honest with their patients about what they will be able to help them do? What do therapists *claim* or *allow patients to believe* in this regard? Which therapists explicitly or implicitly exaggerate the likelihood that they will be able to help their patients make the longed-for changes?

One can find therapists along the whole spectrum from caring, well-meaning, and honest with themselves and their patients to cool, self-centered, self-deceiving, and deceiving and manipulative with their patients. Some think deeply and carefully about what patients want and about their own abilities and limitations. Others operate in a more automatized way, rigidly using their favorite techniques and theories, whether or not they have been shown to help particular kinds of people with particular kinds of problems—or not been shown to help anyone with much of anything. The more caring and conscientious therapists are less likely to misuse whatever diagnostic systems might be available, and the others can probably be counted on to misuse them. A classification system in itself does not have power and ought not to have power. It acquires power because it is produced by one powerful group and used by other powerful ones (such as insurance companies, hospitals, and institutions that grant monies for research), because it is the only game in town, and because it is generally believed to be scientifically based. Most of those features characterize the *DSM*.

Third, should *every* kind of problem that people bring to a therapist be part of a diagnostic classification system? Should loss of one's belief in God, sorrow about the death of a loved one, anxiety about giving a public lecture, worry about gaining weight, belief that the devil is instructing one about how to act, a compulsion to wash one's hands repeatedly, a terror of spiders, a tendency to have nightmares after being in an earthquake, and an intense drive to get straight As in school all be considered appropriate reasons to seek help from a therapist? Who should decide what is appropriate? Should it always be up to the potential patient and therapist to decide? Should we worry that some common, unavoidable problems in living might come to be regarded as signs of mental illness or abnormality if one goes to a therapist for assistance in coping with them? Is it appropriate for a person who has just moved to a new town and has no friends to go to a therapist about a problem in the new job? Is it appropriate for a person who has many friends to go to a therapist about a problem on the job rather than "bother" friends? What about a Native American who is depressed because of having been the butt of racist behavior? Certainly, that person deserves support and help, but how do we balance the risks of that person being labeled "mentally ill" or persuaded that the depression is internally caused against the chances that a therapist could provide the needed assistance? There are no simple answers, and one could ask innumerable questions along these lines, but their relevance to diagnosis as it is practiced today is that a person who sees a therapist for any reason is likely to believe that, or at least wonder whether, something about them is wrong or even "sick" *because* they are seeing a therapist. And the therapist and one's friends and family and co-workers may share that view. After all, it is widely believed that an implication of "being in therapy" is that one needs to be changed or fixed. So it is not enough to say unconcernedly, "Just let everyone with a problem go to a therapist."

Many of the reasons that people end up at therapists' doors are actually very common, though upsetting, problems in their lives, not strange, incomprehensible, or physiologically based conditions, and much trouble comes from the fact that individuals said to have "mental disorders" and "mental illnesses" (discussed in more detail in Chapters 2 and 3) are usually assumed to be qualitatively different from most people. Mentally ill people tend to be considered not just more or less of something than the rest of the population but "other than," different in some puzzling, mystifying way. Some therapists tell me that they don't think in terms of their patients being normal or abnormal, that they simply take the problems the patients present and try to work with them in the ways they think best, and I know this is true for some. However, as will be discussed in detail later on, the *DSM* authors say explicitly that a mental disorder is *not* an "expectable" response to what happens in one's life; thus, they draw a clear line between those whose behavior makes no sense and everyone else. Whether or not it ought to be this way, many therapists and many patients *do* equate abnormality with mental disorder and even with being "in therapy." Some mental health professionals add to the stigmatizing of people called mentally ill by telling stories meant to illustrate how weird and how different from (and inferior to) themselves are their patients or give them offensive nicknames (mental retardation is listed in the *DSM*, and therapists frequently call some mentally retarded children "FLKs," which stands for "funny-looking kids"). Some therapists cast their patients as different from themselves by joining the long tradition of not believing what their patients tell them. It is now well known that Sigmund Freud at first believed women patients who told him they had been sexually abused as children by their fathers or other adult male relatives, but later he announced that there had been no such assaults, that in childhood the little girls had just *wished* to have sex with their fathers. This legacy persists today—again, not for good, caring therapists but for many, and this disbelief is not limited to women patients' descriptions of sexual abuse. As Jeffrey Moussaieff Masson has written, it often extends to anything that patients, especially female ones, might say.

I have been concerned for so long about the disparaging remarks that I have heard some therapists make about patients that I considered writing a book called *What Your Therapist Will Tell Other Therapists But Won't Tell You*. These offensive attitudes toward patients were illustrated at a recent APA convention, where some "psychiatric survivors," former patients in the mental health system, had been invited by the APA to speak at a symposium. Of the thousands attending the convention, only two people showed up to hear the survivors' session, but the huge ballroom down the hall was mobbed with psychiatrists who wanted to hear their colleague, Robert Stolorow, present a slide show about sexual perversions.

Diagnosing people in distancing ways encourages the

use of dramatic interventions, such as psychotropic drugs and electroshock therapy. After all, the weirder the patients seem to be, the more likely it is that uncaring therapists and researchers or those who do not bother to think very carefully will try methods they wouldn't want anyone to use on them. If we think people are very different from us, it is easier to be unaware of their pain. Unfortunately, some of the therapy and research is done by those who are able to ignore the humanness of their patients and research participants.

And Now, the *DSM*

It is not yet possible to develop a classification system for all problems people bring to therapists without running the risk that those problems will all be treated as forms of mental illness. As noted, there has been absolutely no massive, comprehensive, scientifically executed study of the best ways to help people with their various problems. Yet *despite* all of this, the American Psychiatric Association claims to have produced a diagnostic system based on scientific research that will allow us to know what kinds of treatment will be helpful for whom. Much of this book deals with the many respects in which that claim is unwarranted, as well as with the ways that that diagnostic system has been knowingly and unknowingly misused, so that inestimable numbers of people have been harmed.

When I have worked in hospitals and other mental health settings, team heads and clinic directors have told me that I am required to assign a *DSM* diagnosis to each patient but that "it really doesn't matter which one you choose. No one cares anyway." Clearly, some practicing therapists know how little use diagnostic categories are and how little scientific basis there is for them. But it is patently untrue that "no one cares": It matters a great deal to someone whether they are called a Paranoid Personality or an Immature Personality. Often, patients find out—and now have a legal right to know—how they are classified. But the simple fact is that many therapists, as I have seen firsthand, play fast and loose with the categories in the *DSM*, not taking much care to ensure that a patient really fits the criteria for the label that they assign. We then have uncertainty compounding uncertainty: a classification system that was not scientifically developed is claimed by its producers to *be* scientific and also to help produce more scientific research by ensuring that, for instance, all people will be diagnosing "schizophrenia" identically, allowing careful studies to be done. But therapists do not uniformly take care that they call schizophrenic only those people who meet the *DSM* criteria, and this means that the research becomes virtually useless. Furthermore, although the *DSM* authors implied in a 1993 "Fact Sheet" that the *DSM-IV* is "essential" in deciding what treatment a patient needs, their work simply has *not* been about finding out which treatments help people with which kinds of problems. Indeed, their research has been about a far more elementary question—"Are two psychiatrists likely to assign a given patient the same diagnostic label?"—and has yielded very poor results (see Chapter 7). Obviously, if two therapists cannot even agree on a *DSM* diagnosis for a patient, it is not yet possible to know what treatment would help. Do we treat on the basis of therapist A's diagnosis or therapist B's?

In contrast to other therapists, psychiatrists have a disproportionate amount of influence in deciding who is normal, not only because their major association publishes a diagnostic handbook but also because they are medical doctors and are therefore associated with the medical system. As a result, they tend to be accorded higher status.

Psychiatrist Peter Breggin notes that the APA represents thirty-five thousand of the approximately forty thousand American psychiatrists and says, "In recent years APA has developed legislative and promotional departments to increase the power and influence of psychiatry. It spends money to win over the public, the press, and state and federal governments."

The very fact that the APA published a book of diagnoses gives it power, because there are so few competitors. The only other major diagnostic systems are from the Group for the Advancement of Psychiatry (GAP) and the World Health Organization's International Classification of Diseases (ICD). The GAP system was designed to be applied only to children and adolescents and is relatively rarely used; in the massive 865-page *The New Harvard Guide to Psychiatry*, it is mentioned only once in the text and cited in references three times. In contrast, the *DSM* has sixty-one citations in the index and has an entire chapter devoted to it. The ICD system includes both physical and mental "diseases" but gives far more sparse descriptions of its categories than does the *DSM*. The ICD is mentioned in the *Harvard Guide* several times, but the latter book's only chapter on diagnostic classification is almost entirely about the *DSM* and reads much like a publisher's promotional materials for it. In the *Harvard Guide*'s chapter "The Child," the only classification system mentioned is the *DSM*, and in its chapter "Psychiatric Epidemiology," the authors include a section that strongly supports use of the *DSM* and gives the mistaken impression that it is highly scientific. In the words of Kirk and Kutchins, the *DSM*

> contains the official classification system of psychiatric disorders and as such sets the boundaries of the

domain in which psychiatry claims expertise and exclusive authority. The manual specifies the kind of
behaviors and problems for which the profession's
counsel should be sought and its voice heard [and]
. . . is making a claim regarding psychiatry's authority within the broader community.

The fact that the *DSM* enterprise is surrounded by so
much activity makes it seem as though it must be terribly
important: "By developing a massive superstructure consisting of dozens of committees, and involving hundreds
of participants, the Task Force created the illusion that the
development of the manual was the result of an enormous
research effort," note Kirk and Kutchins.[1]

Although psychiatry is not the only profession that
includes some professionals who make damaging and irresponsible decisions about who is normal, psychiatrists
generally have more power and influence because their
status tends to be higher than that of other kinds of psychotherapists. This is partly because they have M.D. degrees, and in nearly all settings in which M.D.s work, they
have more decision-making power than non-M.D.s about
patients' treatment, including their nearly unique legal
power to prescribe drugs and to order patients committed
for treatment against their will. They also tend to be paid
far higher salaries than psychologists, social workers, and
psychiatric nurses. Furthermore, because they are associated with the medical enterprise, they often give the impression of being more scientific than members of the
other disciplines, although only Ph.D. psychologists and
some other therapists with doctoral degrees—among all
mental health professionals—are required to learn about
and conduct original scientific research. And anyone associated with "science" is likely to be assumed to make ob-

jective, scientific judgments, to know absolutely things that the rest of the populace cannot know or understand. Finally, the very fact that the major psychiatric association in North America bothered to publish a book of diagnostic categories adds to the impression that they know more than anyone else about who is not normal and what should be done about that. It is perhaps ironic that the *DSM* was not a response to any groundswell of demand for a classification system from ordinary therapists who do not do research and are not interested in the APA's power politics. In fact, in one study, 55 percent of clinical social workers said that the *DSM* diagnoses did not accurately reflect their clients' problems, and only one-third felt it was helpful for treatment planning. In my twenty-five years in this field, I have rarely met any clinicians who used the *DSM* unless they were required in their workplaces to do so.

In spite of this, the psychiatric establishment has an inordinate influence. Peter Breggin has pointed out, "Unfortunately, since psychiatry dominates the mental health profession, much of what is wrong with psychiatry is also wrong with the whole field." As some mental health professionals believe that, with the *DSM* in hand, they are capable of and justified in deciding who is and who is not normal, the principles embodied in the *DSM* come to permeate our entire culture. I have watched in action many therapists who don't even ask themselves, "Is this person who has come to see me normal or abnormal?" but instead ask themselves only *which* category of abnormality (or "mental disorder," in *DSM* terms) the person fits. Some particularly irresponsible therapists even actively "teach" patients the ways in which they are "sick" (for instance, for "Self-defeating Personality Disorder," "Don't you see how you unconsciously must have *wanted* your spouse to leave you and thereby *made* it happen?"), and patients then both tell others about the nature of their own alleged abnormalities and diagnose them in their friends and family members. *DSM* advocates also spread such dogma when they appear on talk shows or write magazine columns.

So in practice, decisions about who is normal begin with at most a few dozen people—mostly male, mostly white, mostly wealthy, mostly American psychiatrists. This small clique has so much power because they are the architects of the *DSM*. Making the public aware of the way that *DSM* decisions are made is a powerful way to fortify both therapists and the general public against the negative effects such decisions can have. We badly need a demystification of the whole process. This means looking at the shockingly unscientific basis of the *DSM*, the politics and arbitrariness involved in deciding who is normal, and the motives of the major players.

The *DSM* is by no means the only worrying element of current mental health practice. It is simply one distillation of a long and widespread tradition in which prejudices come into play when those with the power to influence others make their decisions about who is and who is not normal. There are serious limitations in the vast majority of North American training programs for all mental health professionals because of the virtual absence of material about women, racialized people, lesbians and gays, and people with disabilities, except to pathologize them.

I hope that if readers learn only one thing from this book, it will be that there is nothing magical about the process of deciding who is and who is not normal and that such decisions must always be carefully questioned. Indeed, when we hear about such a decision being made, the first question to ask should always be, "For what reason are they doing this?" Will the label lead to the labeled person getting more help—help that really works—than if no label were given? And will the label have negative consequences for the person to whom it is applied? In the area of what is usually called mental illness, rarely will labeling really help the labeled person, and nearly always it will have damaging effects. The next question should be, "normal" or "ill/disordered" according to whom? And compared to what standard? Implicit in these questions is the notion that there are many different ways we could decide whom to regard as normal and whom as abnormal.

2

Whose Normality Is It, Anyway?

Some critics wonder if the multiplication of mental disorders has gone too far, with the realm of the abnormal encroaching on areas that were once the province of individual choice, habit, eccentricity or lifestyle.

—Erica Goode, "Sick, or Just Quirky?"

Ask ten people whether the object in the middle of your kitchen is a table, and chances are they will unanimously agree that it is. But ask ten people—even ten therapists—whether any particular person is normal and, if not, *why* they consider the person to be abnormal, and you will almost certainly get a large number of quite different replies. Mental health researchers have conducted research in hopes of proving that therapists can agree on who is normal and who is not (and if not, in what way). But that research revealed that this kind of agreement is in fact extremely rare. To understand how shaky is the *DSM*'s foundation, it is essential to understand that the whole project of trying to define normality always and necessarily involves arbitrary decisions.

Normality Is Not "Real," Like a Table

There is no condition we can absolutely and indisputably call normality, but that fact hasn't stopped many people and organizations from claiming that they do know who is normal and who is not. Later I shall describe how the most powerful arbiters of "normality" too often slot people into categories for politically, economically, and emotionally charged reasons while pretending that they are operating in a solidly scientific way. But, in fact, no matter who is doing the classifying—whether it is the American Psychiatric Association or your best friend—normality is what psychologists call a "construct." This means that there is no clear, "real thing" to which the "normality" label necessarily corresponds. In a sense, at some historical moment, a number of people all saw the first table and then chose or invented a word to name it; but with a construct the name comes first, and then different people choose to apply it to different things. The various people and groups using a construct's name rarely agree completely about how to define the term or what to include in it. Constructs—including "normality"—are nearly always the subjects of long and intense debate.

So, for instance, "intelligence" is a construct. What some people mean by "intelligence" is logical thinking and reasoning ability, what others mean is the ability to learn and remember a lot of facts, and still others insist that musical or athletic ability must be included in any good definition of intelligence. Some people think that an uncreative individual cannot properly be regarded as intelligent, and others strongly disagree. While some psychologists have claimed that each person has more or less of a *single* kind of "thing" they call "g" for general intelligence, others have claimed that intelligence is not unitary but rather is some combination of "things." The word is used in different ways, and no one is really right or wrong about what "intelligence" really is. Instead, people who study "intelligence" debate the pros and cons of using the word to refer to different abilities or combinations of abilities.

The same is true of the construct of normality. In some of my university courses, I have asked students to describe how they decide whether or not someone is normal. In trying to do this, they notice that they can begin either by trying to define it carefully or by trying to think of examples of normality and abnormality and then figuring out what kind of definition would allow them to distinguish the two kinds of examples from each other. Whichever approach they use, they learn that using a construct always involves making *choices*. We choose one definition in preference to another, and we choose to exclude certain items from our definition and to include others. Even if we choose to use the term without worrying about how we ourselves would define it, we thereby choose by default to allow other people to interpret our comments about normality according to the different assumptions *they* make about what the word means.

In light of all of this, it is not surprising that when several people—whether therapists or laypeople—are asked to decide whether or not a particular person is normal, those who say the person is *not* normal often give very different reasons for their decisions. Suppose, for instance, that someone is caught in a hurricane or is the target of repeated sexual abuse as a child and has nightmares during sleep and flashbacks during waking hours about those traumatic experiences. Do we call that person normal? If not, do we call that person abnormal because the majority of people in the world do not have terrifying nightmares and flashbacks? Or do we call her abnormal because *by her own description* she is suffering, and as far as we can tell, she is suffering more than most people suffer? If we think that she is suffering more than the average person, how do we make that judgment? And how much suffering pushes her across the line from normal to abnormal? Does she have to suffer more than 50 percent or 75 percent or 99 percent of the population? Does her suffering have to be of a particular kind? What if she tries to minimize the degree of her suffering because she does not feel she deserves sympathy from others or because she can't bear to think about her pain? How can we find out how much she suffers? Even if she willingly and vividly describes the kind and degree of her suffering, is it possible to decide which of any two people is experiencing more anguish and is thus, perhaps, the more abnormal? Do we consider this person abnormal because she still feels frightened, even though the hurricane is over or her abuser has died and thus the original source of her trouble has vanished? If she fears another natural disaster or incident of abuse, do we say she is normally and healthily on guard or that she is abnormally wasting her time worrying over something that might never happen?

What do we make of the people described by a Toronto general practitioner, who has said that he had boosted dosages of drugs for certain patients when they were under a great deal of stress, but when more cooperative housing became available for them, he was able to cut their dosages in half? Then, when funding for those houses was slashed, his patients were back under increased stress, and "The dosages went back up." Were these people normal or abnormal? Mentally ill or healthy? Did they switch back and forth? Sometimes we can only raise important questions, not answer them. But it is never right to act as though an answer is known when it is not.

As these examples show, in regard to emotions and behavior, the flip side of the construct of psychological normality is the concept of mental illness: Although it shouldn't be this way, in our culture a person considered not to be emotionally normal is pretty much automatically considered mentally ill. And as some psychologists choose to define the construct of intelligence as "whatever intelligence tests measure," ignoring the fact that a few, fallible human beings *choose* what goes on those tests, so many therapists, in effect, define mental illness as "whatever leads people to seek psychotherapy." But many people seek such therapy because they are lonely, sad, anxious, scared, or alienated, and as a result of seeking that help, they may have their original problems compounded or eclipsed by being labeled mentally disordered. What may actually be fairly ordinary feelings and behavior are then renamed *signs of mental disorder*, so that often, no one responds to these emotions and behavior themselves but instead treats them as *signs* of the construct called mental disorder, so they switch the focus to the *presumed* problem. People who are especially unlucky will have therapists who too casually use their label to justify prescribing powerful, possibly dangerous drugs, electroshock treatments, or physical confinement; or they may pronounce that their patients' "disorders" are due to still more unproven constructs, such as their alleged "masochism" or "premenstrual emotional disorder."

When Sigmund Freud found that some women who had been diagnosed as hysterical had been sexually assaulted as children, he theorized a causal connection, that the abuse had led to their physical and emotional problems. He had a choice of describing them as reacting normally to a major trauma or as emotionally deviant in some way. Thus, Freud did not *discover* that they were mentally ill but rather *decided* to give them a label that reeked of emotional abnormality: hysteria. After first announcing the important point that sexual abuse in childhood could cause anguish and suffering, he later produced the appalling theory that the women had *not* been sexually assaulted by male relatives but simply *wished* they had been (the Oedipal/Electra theory).

A quite different way to have dealt with the information would have been to avoid labeling the women as hysterical or neurotic and instead to describe them as having fairly unsurprising reactions to being sexually abused. Had Freud managed somehow to do this, the emphasis would have been on the severity of the real trauma and on the traumatizer's selfishness and his betrayal of the child rather than on Freud's claim that the women had wished to have sex with their abusers. In recent years, large numbers of courageous survivors of sexual abuse have made it clear that child sexual abuse is very common. This has made possible a new focus on how understandable it is to develop powerful ways to cope with major trauma rather than on the alleged abnormality of the sufferer. In trying to help people overcome trauma, this newer approach draws attention to the fact that something truly horrible happened to the person and that she has been trying to cope. This is a strengthening and empowering perspective, in contrast to focusing on how "sick" the woman is and on disbelieving her report of what happened to her. If you are a therapy patient, few experiences are as damaging as not being believed by your therapist.

Both laypeople and mental health professionals too easily forget that the process of defining normality has always involved far more "art" (politics, values, social mores) than science. If a salesman sold us two used cars that rapidly disintegrated, we wouldn't dream of buying a third from him. Why should we be quick to believe new claims about truth and normality when they come from the same mental health institutions that brought us now-discredited concepts? Most people recognize that concepts such as "All women have penis envy, and all men have castration anxiety" used to be regarded as gospel but are now widely regarded as untrue, or at least not universal. These examples come from classical psychoanalysis, but the whole history of psychiatry and psychology is filled with pronouncements of "truths" and "cures" that don't turn out to be what their advocates claimed they were. However, that knowledge about past beliefs has not inoculated us against assuming that whatever the top therapists are *now* presenting as true must indeed be so. The more we understand about how some of the so-called experts make ill-considered decisions about our normality and abnormality, the more quickly will we realize when we are next offered shoddy goods.

Just as people in earlier eras believed that their religious leaders knew the absolute truth about how people should act, so today both laypeople and people within the system tend to believe that high-status mental health professionals really "know" what is normal. Often, mental health professionals make a diagnosis as though they have simply *discovered* what is there and where it should be classified instead of *deciding* what is there and how to pigeonhole it. However, a great deal of research has revealed that whether or not particular people are labeled mentally ill and what diagnoses they are given depends on a large number of variables. With her groundbreaking book, *Women and Madness*, Phyllis Chesler noted that the power to decide who is normal has mainly been in the hands of white men who were disproportionately likely to label women, especially third world women, as psychologically abnormal. Other variables that affect who is called normal include the following: which diagnostic labels have been created and are being used at that time; racial stereotypes; stereotypes about different ways that females and males "ought" to behave; stereotypes about how people of different ages are supposed to act; the socioeconomic class to which the patient belongs; the kind of training the therapist has had and the therapist's internal response to the patient's problems; the interaction between patient and therapist; and whether or not the patient and therapist come from the same cultural background. As we shall see in Chapter 7, therapists' rate of agreement with each other about how to diagnose patients is not very good, even using the much-vaunted *DSM*. Such research makes it crystal clear that decisions about normality and abnormality are filled with biases. Now, if the "experts" rarely agree about whether or not someone is normal—and, even if they agree that a person is mentally ill, often fail to see eye-to-eye about which *kind* of "mental illness" that person has—we must draw one of two possible conclusions. One is that the normal/abnormal dichotomy and the categories of mental illness are pretty useless. The other is that we have no way of knowing which one (or more)—if any—of the "experts" really Knows the Truth.

Historical changes reflect the kaleidoscope of ways that normality can be defined. Hundreds of years ago, people who today might be called "mentally unbalanced" or "mentally ill" were "looked upon as the innocent children of God" and sometimes were even venerated. Later, in the name of religion, many were considered to be possessed by demons and were lashed or burned at the stake. In still later eras, they were variously shackled, put on public display, given some forms of asylum, or sold as slaves. Today, most mental health professionals say that their aim is to *cure* rather than to punish or to exorcise a demon from or to bring shame upon the people they are classifying as "mentally ill," "psychiatrically disordered," or whatever else they use as synonyms for abnormality. However, as noted, the way a person is classified in the mental health system tends to have very little bearing on the kind of treatment given or the likelihood of a "cure." What *has* been shown to matter much more than labeling is the nature of the relationship between the therapist and the person seeking relief from anguish or confusion, a finding that is consistent with Thomas Szasz's observation that "the notion of mental illness is used today chiefly to obscure and 'explain away' problems in personal and social relationships, just as the notion of witchcraft was used for the same purpose from the early Middle Ages until well past the Renaissance."

Because the definition of emotional abnormality has changed so often and so profoundly, huge numbers of people have been flipped from the category of "normal" to the category of "mentally ill"—or vice versa. Louise Armstrong asks, "How could that which millions of Americans had embraced in themselves as being *there*, and spent millions of hours grappling with, wrestling with, struggling to tame, and sometimes—finally—declaring conquered ... suddenly be said never to have been there in the first place?"

The flip side of much ordinary behavior being mistakenly labeled "mentally ill" is what Barbara Johnson has called the fact that "some harm is coded as normal." For instance, as I discuss in Chapter 6, extreme forms of traditionally "masculine" behavior, such as extreme emotional coldness or even violence, have tended to be regarded not as psychiatric disorders or even as problems so much as "real-man" conduct.

Because the precise definition of a construct can vary greatly, so, too, can the emotional impact and images a label can call forth in us. What do *normal* and *abnormal* tend to suggest? Hearing the word *normal* tends to bring to mind any or all of the categories in the left-hand column and *abnormal*, those on the right:

Average; typical	Not average; atypical
As people *should* be	Different from how people *should* be
As nature or God meant people to be	Different from how nature or God meant people to be
As it is least dangerous to be	As it is dangerous to be
Similar to how*ever* we see our*selves*	Different from how we see ourselves
Acceptable	Unacceptable
Morally upright and strong	Morally deficient and weak
Responsible for their actions	Not responsible for their actions
Able to exercise self-control	Unable to exercise self-control
Socially appropriate	Socially inappropriate
Not weird	Weird
In touch with reality	Out of touch with reality
Aware of how they affect others	Unaware of how they affect others
Not tending to make *us* feel frightened or anxious	Tending to make us feel frightened or anxious
Not crazy; sane	Crazy; insane
Able to cope with life	Unable to cope with life

Standard dictionary definitions of *normal* reflect many of these meanings, including "conforming to the standard or the common type; usual; regular; natural . . . approximately average; free from any mental disorder; sane . . . free from disease" (*Random House Webster's College Dictionary*). And *mental health* is defined as "psychological wellbeing and satisfactory adjustment to society and to the ordinary demands of life"; whereas *mental illness* is "any of the various forms of psychosis or severe neurosis." *Mental disorder* and *mental disease* are listed as synonyms for *mental illness,* and according to a parenthetical note, the term *mental illness* didn't even come into general use until between 1960 and 1965.

According to both common usage and dictionary definitions, normality is an either-or proposition rather than a continuum. Although some forms of abnormality are usually considered more alarming than others, if *you* are called abnormal, it may be little comfort to know that some other people are considered even *more* abnormal than you. And although it is possible to classify a bit of behavior rather than a whole person as abnormal, most people worry that *they* as entire people (or most of their behavior) are abnormal once anything about them has been labeled abnormal. For instance, many years ago I worked with children who were diagnosed as "learning disabled," and we used to explain carefully to the children that they were simply having more trouble spelling or doing math than a lot of kids but that that did not mean that they were stupid or crazy or bad people, in other words, that they shouldn't think of themselves as fundamentally different from other kids. We also said that there was nothing weird about the trouble they were having, that most people had such problems at some time or other. Sometimes, our message got through, but often it did not.

Ways to Decide Who Is Normal

Few people who make judgments about normality
bother to think through what they mean by the term, but
every time it is used, some assumption about normality is
being at least implicitly invoked, and I have never found
an assumption about normality/abnormality that was not
worrying or problematic. I have chosen to discuss approaches to normality in terms of what is considered to
be *ab*normal because the book is focused on the *DSM*,
which is all about abnormality.

One could divide different models in many different
ways, but I have found it useful to think in terms of the
infrequency model, the conflict or anxiety model, the delay
or fixation model, the reality-testing model, and the disproportion model. I shall shortly describe these models
and present some of the problems with each, but I want
first to say that I do not recommend adopting any of them,
because I cannot say that I have found it either personally
or professionally useful to classify anyone as normal or
abnormal. When I want to help people, the kinds of questions I have found useful are those such as "Can they think
logically and clearly about what is happening to them?" or
"Does their behavior seem to be motivated by love, fear,
need for power, or hatred?" Classifying people along such
lines has quite different implications and consequences
than using a normal/abnormal dichotomy, and this reveals
a crucial point: Whenever we hear of someone labeling
another person as abnormal, we need to ask *for what purpose* they are making that judgment. Are they trying to
help the person they are labeling, or are they trying to
show they are different from, and better than, that person?
And if their intention is to help, is there any evidence to
suggest that applying an abnormality label will actually
further that intention? Such considerations are important

to keep in mind every time "normality" is being considered. We also need always to ask, "normal compared to whom?" because normality always implies some standard (as in the following examples), and we all would find some standards more fitting than others. For instance, I would not want my physical stamina declared abnormal because it fails to match that of the average teenager, and I don't want an abusive husband's behavior considered normal on the grounds that a large number of men are abusive. Thus, we must always ask not only *What is the standard?* but also *Who is choosing the standard?*

As background for looking at each of the normality models, it is helpful to think of criteria for normality as relatively objective or relatively subjective. For instance, some people would use the somewhat objective criterion of "a history of being able to do productive work and support oneself and to form and maintain close relationships"; whereas others would use a more subjective guideline such as "not feeling much distress or inner conflict" as hallmarks of normality. But although it is somewhat easier to assess the first than to know for certain what is going on inside a person, some subjectivity is involved in judging even the former: Different people would make different assessments of what is productive work or a close relationship. Both relatively objective and relatively subjective criteria present other problems. Objective criteria can mask internal conflict and anguish, since some individuals skillfully maintain their work lives and even hold marriages together but at great cost to their peace of mind. Some commonly used subjective criteria may not be sufficient for deciding who is abnormal, since few people would want to classify as normal a serial killer who might feel little anxiety, guilt, or inner conflict. Furthermore, some people who would be called "out of touch with reality" because they consider themselves to be Jesus Christ or the Virgin Mary appear to feel little or no anxiety once they become immersed in believing in their exalted identity, yet most individuals would choose to call them abnormal.

At the heart of all of the basic questions about normality we shall find we are spinning our wheels. There is inevitably a circular process, because in order to think about and study normality, first we have to choose how to define it. Once we have defined it, then we can set about finding ways to measure its properties. But it is hard to find reliable, informative ways to measure aspects of human behavior and emotions, so we encounter a whole host of problems in trying to do the measuring task. Even if we could surmount all of those problems, where would that leave us? We would have found some way to assess who is normal, but that would not prove that we had defined normality "correctly" in the first place, since there is no such thing as a right or wrong definition of normality. Definitions of constructs can be more or less *useful* or can attract greater or fewer numbers of supporters, but they cannot be correct or incorrect. So, for instance, suppose that we choose an *infrequency* model, defining abnormality as what is unusual and normality as what is average. But then we must ask, Average what? Average amounts of happiness? Of anxiety? Of motivation to get good grades in school or to be a good cook? Of courage to try new things? And if we could find some reasonable way to *measure* how happy people are, suppose we find that most people are pretty unhappy and therefore the average person is unhappy or the average family has problems? Do we really want to say that unhappiness is normal? If, on the other hand, we do not choose to define normal as "average" or "most common," then we are plunged immediately into making value judgments, deciding how normal people *ought* to act and feel, deciding which less-common-than-average group is normal. And if value judgments are going to be made, to whom shall we entrust the power to make them?

Another way to think about normality is to call it the *absence of most conflict and anxiety*. But once we call it that, how do we judge who fits the description? As mentioned, we can observe people and *surmise* that they feel conflicted and anxious, but we cannot always make such judgments accurately just by looking. We can *ask* people how they are feeling, but if they tell us they feel anxious, how shall we decide whether the amount of anxiety they feel takes them across the line that divides normal from abnormal? Then, too, the *causes* of conflict and anxiety can change over time as society and culture change. For instance, in the 1950s, men who wished to stay home and take care of their children and women who wished to obtain paid employment were more likely than people today to feel anxiety and conflict caused by social forces urging them in the opposite directions. If what seems "normal" according to this model will change from one historical period and one culture to another, then honest users of the model will make it clear that they cannot designate people as normal or abnormal with certainty or stability, that "normal" is not absolute and forever.

The conflict and anxiety approach has worrying implications when it comes to trying to help people solve their problems. Not long ago, I read a newspaper story about a psychiatric hospital that had started some self-help groups for widows and others for widowers. The nurse in charge said that the groups had helped widows survive their grief but had not been helpful to widowers. She and her co-workers had dealt with that discovery by sending widows to talk to the men who had lost their spouses, and *that,* they found, *was* successful. The men couldn't help each other, but each woman could help a man. The men apparently felt no anxiety about their inability to help each other, so that inability did not come to be considered a problem. In this way, the men's *learned* style of dealing with disturbing feelings by getting sympathy and support from women was perpetuated rather than, say, the mental health experts believing that it might be emotionally healthier for the men to learn to give support to and receive it from members of their own sex. Instead, use of the conflict and anxiety model helped strengthen the notion that both men and women should (normally) look to women for nurturance.

A third way to think about normality is in terms of a *delay or fixation* model. If we think that all well-adjusted people follow a particular course of emotional development, then anyone who seems to be functioning at a stage that is "too young" for their age may be considered abnormal. In the personality theories of many thinkers in the Western Hemisphere, independence and autonomy are the be-all and end-all of psychological development: the older you get, the more independent and separate you are supposed to be and to *want* to be. By this standard, both those men who care deeply about relationships and the majority of women—who have been taught that they *should* care a lot about relationships—have been considered to be underdeveloped or "fixated" at an immature level. Similarly, due to Freud's claim that heterosexuality represents a more advanced level of development than homosexuality, adult homosexuals have often been labeled as delayed at an immature stage of development, as being fixated rather than simply as differing in some respects from heterosexuals.

To use this kind of approach, we need to know if there

is a normal pattern of stages, and the research about this has been deeply flawed and roundly criticized. The criticisms are of two sorts: One is that the research is often sloppy or filled with bias; for instance, in some major research projects, only males were observed but then conclusions were drawn about what is normal for both sexes, so that girls' and women's development seemed inferior. The other kind of criticism is that such research must be based on at least one assumption about what *normal* means. For instance, if we tried to find out how people normally develop, how would we decide what to study? Would we investigate how they usually develop, or how they developed if they have held down the same full-time job for twenty years, or how they developed if they are now able to take moderate risks and to tolerate change well, or how they developed if they have become skilled at resolving problems in their relationships with others, or how they developed if they cannot form close relationships but are terrific at tolerating long periods of time on their own? In other words, this kind of model involves circular reasoning: First, we decide how to define normal development, then we do some research to find out who develops that way, and finally we call "abnormal" anyone who "gets stuck" at a "lower" stage, according to our own choice of definitions of "normal." In its circularity, this model is no different from *all* models of normality, because each begins with a decision about what the word *normal* will be used to signify. After that, it becomes simply a question of finding ways to *measure* the anxiety, the particular kind of development, or whatever else has been chosen as the key sign.

A fourth model of normality is the *reality-testing* one. According to this approach, the better you are at "knowing" what is real, at being "in touch with" reality, the more likely we are to describe you as normal. But first we have to define "reality," and here more problems arise. Whom do we want to define reality for us? This is problematic because, although most people would say that a person who says she is the Virgin Mary is clearly out of touch with reality, others would say that she should not be called abnormal but is only expressing in vivid metaphor her psychospiritual crisis. The dilemma becomes even worse when we have to confront such questions as "Is an interracial couple who decide to have a child out of touch with reality, since they are not regarding as insuperable the problems of racism and ostracism that their child will encounter?" or "Is an ardent feminist who is working for social change out of touch with reality, because she doesn't seem to realize how powerful are the forces that oppose her efforts?" Since some people would think that the problems of racism or the power of anti-equality forces are insuperable, but others would disagree, what is the reality in such cases?

As these examples make clear, a reality-testing model is invariably linked to the question of how reality is defined, and the people who have the greatest power to impose their views of reality on others are those who are most likely to uphold the majority views of reality and normality. Thus, for instance, the traditional therapists who ran the self-help groups for widows and widowers did not choose to declare the men out of touch with reality because they considered men unable to help each other. Like most people in powerful positions, these therapists had a conservative view of reality; accordingly, they assumed the emotionally constricted men to be normal, and they rearranged their environment for them. In a famous 1970 study by psychologist Inge Broverman and her colleagues, therapists described emotionally healthy women as more passive than men, so that a passive man is more likely to be considered out of touch with the reality of being male than is an aggressive man. Similarly, a woman who is upset about a social system that will not allow her to express legitimate anger (because it is unfeminine to do so) is often described as unable to accept "reality" by adapting to her prescribed role. Until recently, a woman who chose not to have a child was considered disturbed, to be denying her femaleness and thereby out of touch with the reality of her biological destiny. Acknowledging that she had a womb was not enough to prove that she was in touch with reality; she had to fill it with a fetus. As these examples show, the criterion of "reality testing" changes over time. It also varies from one culture to another, since the way an inner-city mother might have to think and act in order to protect her children from both police and gang violence would be quite different from the way a mother in a suburb less plagued by such violence might be free to think and act.

A fifth normality model is the *disproportion* model, according to which we are abnormal if we have "too much" or "too little" of some feeling or psychological force. An obvious subtype of this model is the *deficiency* model; that is, a person who has, for example, less self-confidence or intelligence or self-control than some chosen standard is considered abnormal. Some of the problems with this approach are familiar. First of all, how do we find out—or decide—which amounts of which psychological factors are normal? In our definition, need we take into account every conceivable feeling, thought, attitude, or action? How could we decide how much of each factor is necessary for normal functioning? Here again, we confront the two problems of social-historical change and of the need to make value judgments. In the following examples, both of these problems are reflected. If we decided to define normality by a vote, and the majority voted in 1950 that a normal woman is sexually passive but has a powerful sense of duty and poor self-esteem, by 1990 a vote would have yielded a very different picture of the normal woman. Within a single historical period, what the majority of Greek-Americans or African-Americans consider to be normal expressions between male friends is likely to diverge a great deal from what British-Americans consider normal. If the kinds and amounts of psychological factors required for "normality" change from one time to another and from one culture to another, what can the concept mean except what the majority—or the most powerful—believe is appropriate? The proportions considered normal are in a state of constant flux. If they were not, it would be obvious to everyone who was and who was not normal.

All of these models are *difference* models, because they are various frameworks for focusing on differences between people who will henceforth be considered normal and people who will not. Writing about the effects of labeling some human beings as different from the rest of us, progressive psychiatrist Matthew Dumont implies that we should not assume that labeling is well left to the mental health "experts":

> To be mentally ill is to feel one's membership in society up for question. It is to be marginal, deviant. A mental health clinic cannot be expected to function as a model of utopia, but it can at least try to minimize the forces of alienation and mute the discords of a society that is endlessly exclusive. These are not the technical issues of psychotherapy or medical management; they are human ones.

Clearly, the project of trying to define normality is extremely problematic. There seems to be no very good way to do it and certainly no way that doesn't involve sweeping value judgments, virtually insurmountable definitional and research problems, and serious dangers to those who are classified as abnormal. Unfortunately, the people who put together the *DSM* do not appear to have grappled much with most of these concerns. The terms *normal* and *abnormal* do not appear in their glossary, but by the third edition of *DSM* they had preceded their definition of *mental disorder* by saying that they make "no assumption that each category of mental disorder is a completely discrete entity with absolute boundaries dividing it from other mental disorders or from no mental disorder." This disclaimer appears to be an attempt to justify whatever arbitrary, subjective, and biased choices they make about whom to classify as disordered. It is disturbing that, following their acknowledgment that there is no such thing as a discrete state called "mentally disordered," separate from the state of not being mentally disordered, one finds an entire book of details that are purported to teach us exactly how to recognize not only when disorder is present but also precisely which kind of mental disorder it is. As Kovel has written, the *DSM* follows the pattern of Linnaeus, who named species and distinguished them from each other because he believed that there *were* such things as species. If the *DSM* authors do not believe there is a clearcut state of mental disorder, they should not claim to be able to make fine distinctions among subtypes of this nonexistent entity. If they do not believe in it, it seems that their claim that mental disorders are not discrete entities would appear to be a disingenuous attempt to ward off their critics.

Apparently, in 1975 the folks working on what would become the *DSM-III* tried to come up with a definition of *mental disorder*, but "only one member was able to actually attempt a definition, and it apparently wound up winding back and around itself, ending up in the neighborhood of the laboriously loquacious and abstruse." Then, *DSM-III* chief Robert Spitzer and a colleague came up with a definition that included the statement "Mental disorders are a subset of medical disorders," a claim that is, quite simply, unsubstantiated. Calling mental disorders a subset of medical disorders was a daring but productive political move, because it gives the former the appearance of being scientifically proven and indisputably true, in the way that there is rarely any question about whether or not someone has a medical disorder such as high blood pressure or cancer. As Louise Armstrong has observed, once medical-scientific language is used to talk about emotional or behavioral issues, "many citizens will begin believing they know what they are talking about when they are actually speaking in tongues."

The definition of *mental disorder* in the *DSM-IV* reads as follows:

> a *clinically significant behavioral or psychological syndrome or pattern* that occurs in an individual and that is associated with *present distress* (e.g., a painful symptom) or *disability* (i.e., *impairment* in one or more *important* areas of functioning) or with a significantly increased risk of suffering death, pain, disability, or an important loss of freedom. In addition, this syndrome or pattern *must not be merely an expectable and culturally sanctioned response* to a particular event, for example, the death of a loved one. Whatever its original cause, it must currently be considered a manifestation of a behavioral, psychological, or biological dysfunction in the individual. Neither deviant behavior . . . nor conflicts that are primarily between the individual and society are

mental disorders unless the deviance or conflict is a symptom of a dysfunction in the individual. [my italics]

There is a host of problems embodied in that definition. First of all, every italicized phrase allows enormous scope for subjectivity and bias. Who decides whether or not someone's behavior or feelings are "clinically significant"? Since some degree of distress is an inevitable part of life, who decides what is a sufficiently high level of distress to be considered part of a mental disorder? Who decides what constitutes an impairment in functioning, and who decides which areas of functioning are important enough to be implicated in a mental disorder? In a sense, the most alarming phrase is that the pattern must not be "merely an expectable . . . response to a particular event." The most humane, thoughtful, and effective therapists that I know believe that the most important part of much treatment is the therapist's attempt to understand how the patient feels and what led to that feeling. To state the problem in its most extreme (and admittedly, somewhat exaggerated form), in giving someone a *DSM* diagnosis, a therapist must believe that the patient thinks and feels in ways that are qualitatively different from those of most human beings, since by definition their responses cannot be "expectable." This attitude, which I have not infrequently observed, is cold and inhumane. Furthermore, it does not help anyone feel better except therapists who thereby convince themselves that they are better people than their patients. One must also ask, "How do we decide what is 'expectable'?" If we define it as statistically likely, we encounter the problems discussed earlier with an infrequency model. And how infrequent must a response be to make it unexpectable—one person in one hundred responds this way, one in one thousand, one in a million? Who should choose the cutoff point? If there is no obvious, statistically compelling cutoff point, whom shall we trust to assess what is expectable?

Every category of mental disorder in the *DSM* is a construct, just as much as "normality" and "mental disorder" are constructs. One of the most glaring illustrations of this fact is the history of the treatment of homosexuality in various editions of the manual. After listing it as a mental disorder, the APA announced in 1974 that it would remove it for *DSM-III*. The APA's vote showing 5,854 members supporting and 3,810 opposing its removal is one manifestation of the fact that this "mental disorder" is a construct. The claim that it would be deleted turned out to be completely untrue, because *DSM-III* included "ego dystonic homosexuality," which essentially means being homosexual and not feeling fully comfortable about it—hardly a surprising consequence of being lesbian or gay in our culture but surely not a mental illness. Every *DSM* category requires that the therapist make subjective judgments, and naturally there are some therapists to whom we would more happily entrust such judgments than others. The problem is that, when people are in distress and seeking help, they rarely have much time to find out whether their therapist deserves such trust before the labels of abnormality are assigned. Then, too, the *DSM*'s inclusion of distress as part of their definition of disorder carries with it all of the problems described earlier. Trying to decide whether a person's functioning is "impaired" involves the difficulties about trying to judge objectively whether or not someone's ability to work or to have relationships is normal. In summary, there is wide scope for subjectivity and bias in the *DSM*'s definition of mental abnormality.

The one potentially good aspect of the *DSM* definition

is the note that one should not diagnose a mental disorder primarily because the individual is in conflict with society. However, it is all very well to say that, but as officials of the American Psychiatric Association in general and the *DSM* authors in particular have acknowledged, they have absolutely no way to ensure that in actual practice, psychiatrists and other physicians and therapists actually follow that principle.

We shall not here resolve the question of what the definition of normal *should* be or even if we ought to try to divide the world into the normal and the abnormal, but we must never forget that there are always reasons, based on a wide variety of honorable and dishonorable motives, whenever someone makes such a decision. I honestly don't yet know whether I believe that any benefit comes from "abnormality" or "mental illness" being used as part of a dichotomous labeling system. But one way to understand and explore those issues, as well as to assess whether the negative real-life consequences of labeling are worth enduring for some greater good, is to understand *how* those with the most power to declare who is not normal make their decisions.

The question "Can we really know who is normal?" is a specific case of the general question "Can we ever really know the Truth?" or even "Is there such a thing as Truth?" I won't, of course, be addressing that larger debate, because the focus of this book is that the *DSM* authors *unjustifiably claim* that through scientific research they have found the Truth about normality and abnormality, including effective, helpful treatments and cures. But although that is my focus here, I must confess that I often wonder whether not only many psychiatrists but also many mental health professionals of all kinds think there is such a thing as a normal, healthy person.

I end this chapter with former "mental patient" Judi

Chamberlin's observation about the profundity of issues related to the topic of normality/abnormality:

> The question What is mental illness? leads directly to some of the major philosophical questions with which the human race has grappled throughout history: What is the mind? What is the relationship between the brain and the mind? These questions are far too important to be left to the psychiatrists, whose medical-school training is largely irrelevant to dealing with them. By their training, psychiatrists have already made the assumption that mental illness exists as a counterpart to physical illness.

3

Do Mental Health Professionals Think Anyone Is Normal?

The history of mental health care is a vacillating mix of the aberrant and the rational that is equal to anything displayed by the unfortunates who require the care. Mythology, morality, medicine, pragmatism, politics and pills have all been—and still are—components of the system's evolutionary pendulum.

—John Marshall, *Madness*

Before looking at the way the *DSM* producers go about deciding who is normal, a more basic issue needs to be addressed: Do mental health professionals think *anyone* is normal? This is not just a tongue-in-cheek question, a rhetorical device that illustrates my concern about the free-and-easy way so many therapists brand huge numbers of people as abnormal, for psychotherapists who see abnormality everywhere are not as rare as one would wish. In fact, it has been said that "a normal family is one that has not yet been assessed clinically."

The histories of psychoanalysis, psychiatry, and many schools of psychology have largely been histories of attempts to understand what is *wrong* with people, even if some of the work from those fields has then been used to try to explain "normal" development. Although it is important to try to understand what can go wrong, both professionals and laypeople tend to look *exclusively* at problems and weaknesses. This masks crucial parts of the pictures of people's lives, and it also skews therapy, so that we don't much look for strengths on which patients can build. The focus on pathology has been so influential that cocktail party chatter often includes remarks such as that certain dream-images are phallic symbols and, therefore, signs of penis envy in women or castration anxiety in men; that everyone's parents (usually mothers) messed them up emotionally; that there is no such thing as a healthy family; and so on. The preoccupation with problems, weaknesses, and strangeness works like a detour sign, streaming the traffic of clinical interpretation toward abnormality. As mentioned, interpretations veer more sharply away from normal when the prospective patient is poor, relatively uneducated, a member of a racialized group, a member of an age, ethnic, or cultural group different from that of the therapist, and so on. When I was an undergraduate at Harvard/Radcliffe in the late 1960s, a much-loved professor named Robert White was considered remarkable because his work as a psychologist was about people who were considered normal—how they behaved and felt, how they had developed, what they wanted to do. Psychologist Henry A. Murray, who is known as the father of clinical psychology, had retired by the time I was in college, but his richly textured work on normal human functioning provided fascinating material. Unfortunately, such psychologists are still few in number.

As a perceptive woman who spent years as a patient on a psychiatric hospital service told me, "If you go to a therapist, they can only give you what they have. They have a certain kit of tools with which to work—and I happen to think it is a pretty empty bag." Perhaps, I would say, not so much empty as too much filled with forms of abnormality. The prestigious *New Harvard Guide to Psychiatry* has no listing for "normality" in its index, and with two exceptions (Nicholi and Nemiah), the authors of the thirty-six chapters write as though there is no need to try to define "abnormality" or to specify how it differs from normality.

I noticed years ago, when I began my own training as a therapist at the age of twenty-two and was suddenly expected both to help people and to know more about them than they knew about themselves, that I felt quite daunted and insecure. Like most therapists-in-training, I dealt with those feelings by turning to my teachers and to books and articles about therapy in order to learn what I ought to do, what was the "truth" about how to help people. I found most of my teachers to be preoccupied with people's weaknesses and abnormalities to the exclusion of their strengths and abilities, and the same was true of the authors of the books and articles we were told to read. They seemed to consider it more serious to fail to see existing problems than to see psychopathology when it was not there, although in fact the consequences of either can be damaging. Frankly, it took a great deal of experience and support from people I respected to be able to go beyond my own persistent search for abnormality in people who came to me in need. When I read the half-serious, half-humorous book *Games Analysts Play* and came across material like the following, it didn't seem very different from what I had heard from quite a few therapists of many kinds. Describing a game they call Opposites, authors Shepard and Lee present these brief dialogues:

> (1) P[atient]: I really love my wife.
>   T[herapist]: It seems to me that you are trying to hide the fact that you hate her.
> (2) P: My mother was terrible and I hated her.

T: Perhaps what you are really trying to tell me
is that you loved her too much.

Since 1979, as I have worked with psychology, psychiatry,
and social work students and interns, I have had to spend
a lot of time trying to counteract the pressures placed on
them throughout most of their training to seek out and
focus on the pathology in people. Added to the common
emphasis on what is *wrong* with people, we now have a
massive *DSM-IV*, listing fully 374 different ways to be
mentally ill, up from 297 in the previous edition. This
listing is extremely influential even though, as Kirk and
Kutchins say in their book, *The Selling of DSM*, "There
is little agreement among mental health experts that disorders can be easily or clearly separated from nondisorders."
When there is no clear demarcation between normal and
abnormal, it is all the more unlikely that therapists will often
classify people as normal. Still another force that points
therapists' attention toward the abnormal is the common practice of looking *only* within the individual for
the source of problems. This renders it unlikely that
therapists will consider such factors as poverty, racism, or
ageism in trying to understand why a patient might be
depressed. They are more likely to probe exclusively for
signs that their patients enjoy suffering, set impossibly
high standards of achievement for themselves, or have
negative self-concepts. Working with a patient only along
these lines is wrongheaded when social influences are ignored, and it certainly increases the risk of teaching the
patient self-blame and shame when these are not appropriate or health-promoting. Historically, social workers
have been more inclined to take social factors into account
in trying to assist unhappy people, but as social worker
Ben Carniol has pointed out, even their profession has

been turned toward a focus on individuals' intrapsychic sources of trouble. This has been partly because social work has been influenced by psychiatry and psychology and partly because some social workers who feel powerless to eradicate poverty and other social ills find it less upsetting to act as though the problems come from within the individual.

Naturally, when people come seeking help and saying, "I am miserable," one does not deny their unhappiness or refuse to try to help them understand and overcome their problems. But these goals are harder to achieve when one focuses virtually exclusively on what is presumably *wrong* with them. When, for instance, trainees under my supervision conducted assessments of children who were doing badly in school, whether or not they found that a child had a reading or spelling problem, they always made an effort to identify the child's strengths and abilities as well. That yielded a more accurate and complete assessment, for after all, none of us is composed solely of our weaknesses, and it also gave the child's teachers something with which they could work, rather than just an *absence* of, say, reading achievement in the child. At the end of the assessment we could look at the children, who knew they were in our clinic because they were having trouble, and say, "Yes, you are having trouble with X, but you do Y really well, and we are also very impressed by how hard you work."

Experience with women survivors of incest has shown that when therapy groups focus constantly and solely on the incest itself, survivors have far more trouble overcoming their anguish, shame, and fear than when the groups also include some attention to the women's strengths, interests, and aims. When the latter approach is neglected, the survivor can come to feel that her whole identity is that of an incest victim, and the chances that she will attempt suicide increase. This is not to say that she does not need to spend *some* time focusing on the devastating experiences but only that an exclusive focus on them can be frankly harmful.

Therapists' tendency to look for problems was dramatically illustrated in a classic study by Maurice Temerlin and William Trousdale, who wrote about "the social psychology of clinical diagnosis," the effect of suggestion on whether clinicians believe they are looking at psychopathology. This is an extremely important issue, because when one is a therapist and a potential patient walks in, that very situation "suggests," tends to encourage one to see, psychopathology rather than normality or simply problems in living. This tendency is caused not only by therapists' training and expectations but also by their tendency to urge each other to look for abnormality. One seems to have more expertise if one diagnoses pathology in a patient than if one says there is nothing wrong. In a recent court case in which I was involved, the social worker and psychologist at a community mental health clinic decided that a woman was quite paranoid and unreasonably belligerent, and the child welfare workers pretty much accepted the clinic staff's description of her. Finally, the woman went to see a private psychologist, who found her in the first interview to be an expressive, emotionally intense, but believable and reasonable person. Then, that psychologist talked with the clinic and child welfare staff and totally reversed her view of the woman. Although such changes can be justified when they result from one professional giving new information to another, they can also be unjustified when they result from the kinds of social/ professional pressure to which people sometimes respond by accepting their colleagues' views as their own.

Back to the Temerlin and Trousdale study. These researchers wrote a script of a diagnostic interview in which the person being interviewed established a warm relationship with the interviewer, talked coherently about his feelings and thoughts, was able to recall childhood memories clearly, was emotionally expressive without overdoing it, and was free from such problems as hallucinations, grandiosity, depression, or disorganized thinking. They had a professional actor enact the script in a way that was intended to show that he had no psychological problems but was intellectually curious about therapy, and they taped him being interviewed as though he were a prospective therapy client. It is not unusual for people to make appointments to see therapists and begin by asking if there is something wrong with them—not what but if. After all, there is so much talk about emotional problems and abnormality that many people wonder if they need help. If they don't feel particularly upset, they wonder if they may have problems they haven't recognized.

Temerlin and Trousdale showed the tape to undergraduate students, advanced law students, graduate students in clinical psychology, practicing clinical psychologists, and practicing psychiatrists. The psychologist who showed the undergraduates, clinical psychology students, and psychologists the tape remarked casually that the person on the tape "looked neurotic but actually was quite psychotic." The law students were given the same suggestion by the instructor in their law school course, and the psychiatrists were told that two psychiatry Board members, one of whom was a psychoanalyst, had listened to the tape and had agreed that the man looked neurotic but was actually psychotic. All participants were asked to indicate how the interviewee should be classified, choosing from a list that included various mental disorders, personality types, *and* the category *normal or healthy personality*. Then they were asked to describe the patient briefly, sticking to a description of the person's actual behavior and avoiding clinical inferences, abstract concepts, or technical terms: "Simply state what you actually heard—actually observed—this person say and do." After writing their reports, participants were given the chance to change their original diagnosis if they wished.

After one psychologist told the researchers he diagnosed four extremely serious mental disorders in this man because the fellow looked normal but "normal people do not come into a clinic," the researchers decided to recruit three additional groups. One diagnosed the man based on the same tape in a clinical setting but after hearing the prestigious person say that the patient "looked like a normal, healthy man." A second diagnosed the man from the same interview with no prior suggestion at all but in a clinical setting, and the third group diagnosed outside a clinical setting, without prior suggestion, ostensibly helping to select engineers and scientists to work in industry. The third group was told this was a "personnel interview" designed to see if the candidate was employable for a research corporation. The tape was changed for this last group only in that the interviewee did not express curiosity about psychotherapy.

Not a single member of any of the last three groups diagnosed the man as psychotic, but significant numbers of the first five groups did, and most in the first five who did not say he was psychotic said he was neurotic. Most people in the control groups said either that he was healthy and normal or that he had "mild adjustment problems," but only tiny percentages of the people in the first groups (and in fact no psychiatrists at all) used either of those categories. Real-life situations can correspond to either the control-group or the experimental-group ones: The control-group ones are similar to therapists being asked if a patient has psychological problems *without* being told that someone believes she or he does, and the experimental-group ones are typical of what happens in clinical settings, where one is asked to see patients because they themselves or other people suspect that something is wrong with them. This study demonstrates clearly the way many therapists are influenced by their colleagues to look for the abnormal.

A similar outcome of a study by some of the *DSM* bigwigs themselves was recently reported. When they asked therapists to assign diagnoses to both patients and nonpatients, Janet Williams, Robert Spitzer, and a large group of their colleagues found that the therapists assigned *DSM* diagnoses to more than one-quarter of the *nonpatients*.

An especially worrying practice that is on the increase is to assume that a patient who has a physical problem such as stomach pain or persistent fatigue *must* have a mental disorder if physicians haven't identified a physiological cause. A particularly tragic case that was reported in every major Canadian publication resulted in the death of a young boy who was admitted to a Toronto hospital with repeated vomiting. At one point, when no physical problem that might cause the vomiting had been found, a psychiatric consultation was requested. The outcome of that consultation was an assertion that the vomiting was psychologically caused and a recommendation that the staff make the child clean up his own vomit as a way of teaching him to stop. The young boy died soon afterward and was found to have a bowel blockage.

In a less tragic but still worrying example, a woman I had known for several years went to Mexico on a vacation and contracted a digestive problem that persisted after her return home. A physician treated her with medication, and her severe diarrhea stopped, but she continued to have difficulty swallowing food without becoming nauseated. She had been in therapy for some time, and her psychiatrist informed her that the nausea was caused by her intense anxiety. I said that she seemed no more anxious now than she had during all the time I had known her, and I suggested that she try some Maalox in case the infection she had developed in Mexico had left her digestive tract irritated. Fortunately, she tried the Maalox before going on the tranquilizers her therapist wanted to prescribe, and after one dose her nausea vanished. Too often, doctors who are reluctant to say, "I don't know what is causing this problem," say instead, "You have a psychological disorder." This practice is not limited to psychiatrists and other physicians, for psychologist Susie Orbach claimed in her book *Fat Is a Feminist Issue* that women put on weight because they do not want to be treated as sex objects. I am certainly a feminist, but although some women probably do gain weight for the reason Orbach suggests, I know from my own experience that many women who are described as overweight are only classified that way because of our culture's obsession with thinness for women, and some women who easily gain weight and lose it with difficulty have digestive disorders or other physical problems.

Ironically, many so-called mental disorders are increasingly assumed to have physical bases. Szasz has said, "Respectable scientists have been interested only in afflictions of the body," and so, in order to enhance their professional status, those who dealt with "problems of human living" have treated them "as though they were manifestations of physical illnesses." The *DSM* editions have promoted this approach generally, because they are produced by a medical association and because of the use of the term *disorder*. J. L. T. Birley has pointed out that, in recent *DSM*s, the word *disease* was replaced by the word *disorder* and opined that this makes little difference, except to increase the likelihood that increasing numbers of trivial conditions will be included. The *DSM-IV* intensified the approach further by omitting a category called Organic Mental Disorder because "it incorrectly implied that other psychiatric disorders did not have biological contribution." This implies that everything listed as a mental disorder in the handbook has a biological contribution, a patently unfounded claim. Furthermore, now that biomedical approaches—looking for physical causes and prescribing drugs for emotional problems—are so prevalent and so energetically promoted by psychiatrists and drug companies, emotional "abnormality" often seems even more hopeless and permanent. Describing herself as a former "mental patient," Judi Chamberlin has written that psychiatrists' classification of patients as suffering from "depression," a label that frequently leads to prescription of drugs or electroshock therapy, often stands in the way of their doing what she feels they need to do, which is to become aware of their feelings. (Ironically, antidepressants can mask feelings and can also *cause* depression.)

Some therapists are far better than others, of course. There are those who say outright that they wish to help people get through "normal" but difficult periods in life, such as losing a job, going through a divorce, or losing a child. And some people who describe themselves as feminist therapists or lesbian-positive therapists, for instance, say explicitly that they aim to help people who have suffered because of sexist or homophobic treatment, *not* to label such people as abnormal and in need of repair. (Not all therapists who make such claims actually stick closely to their principles in the course of therapy, but some do.)

But even the patients of well-intentioned therapists often consider themselves to be seriously damaged, deficient, or otherwise abnormal. This is partly because therapy tends to involve either some work on feelings that our society considers negative, such as anger, shame, or fear, or the attribution of blame to the patient's mother (or, less often, the patient's father), or both. So the patient feels grotesque for having feelings that seem bad or strange and also feels damaged by having been raised by such a horrid mother. Patients also consider themselves abnormal or deficient partly because therapy is widely regarded as a place where one goes in order to be fixed, made whole, untwisted. As I know from my own practice, as well as from other therapists' and patients' reports, unless a therapist takes great care continually to deal with these issues in depathologizing ways, simply being in therapy can tend to make the patient *feel* abnormal.

We have Sigmund Freud to thank for a rather curious state of affairs. He claimed to know that all children everywhere want to have sex with the parent of the other sex and that all girls and women enjoy suffering. Since these claims became so widely accepted in our culture, and since Freud asserted that these feelings were universal, they came to seem "normal" in the sense of typical or even inescapable, even though they certainly sounded strange to most of us. Then, shockingly, because of the power and influence that therapists subscribing to these notions have had over their individual patients and the general public, these feelings came to seem *not* strange. In fact, in some circles—especially some highly intellectual ones—still today, if you do not "admit" to having such feelings, you are thought to be weird or at least to be unduly defensive. Even what may seem truly bizarre and what is unsupported by any evidence or real logic comes in this way to seem universal, inevitable, and, in that sense, normal. In his novel *1984*, George Orwell called this Doublethink, and his readers have found it frightening. So should we wherever we find it, for this is how we come to see abnormality in everyone.

A current example of Doublethink about normality is the way many mental health professionals classify behavior in old people. I have heard therapists say matter-of-factly that in old people, withdrawal, depression, and apathy are normal. Surely no one would accept such a claim about young people; the fact that it has been widely accepted when applied to old people merely reflects our society's biased belief that if misery in old age is normal, then we needn't think about or try to alleviate it. It also reflects most people's willingness to believe whatever they are told about a group to which they do not belong, especially if it makes their own seem superior. But although withdrawal, depression, and apathy are unsurprisingly *common* in a culture that pulls away from, devalues, and withholds resources and involvement and activities from old people, do we want to call that *normal*? Robert Butler's prize-winning book *Why Survive? Being Old in America* was necessary to propose an idea then considered surprising— that old people may actually want to stay connected to people they love and do not necessarily long to withdraw from society. A related manifestation of strange assumptions about normality in aging people is that in many nursing homes and hospitals it is considered normal to speak to old people in patronizing tones or to speak in front of them as though they were not present, according to social worker Rachel Josefowitz Siegel. Implicit in such conduct is that the old person normally does not mind. But not to mind such treatment is surely, by any sense of the word, not normal, healthy, or growth-enhancing. In this way,

vast numbers of people are first made unhappy, deperson-
alized, or otherwise badly treated as a result of stigmatiza-
tion and devaluation in our culture; then their behavior
comes to show the negative effects of such mistreatment;
and finally the culture rather sweepingly deems that disturbing but now-common behavior to be normal because
it is average, "part of the normal course of aging."

Patterns similar to that with respect to aging are found
in assumptions about normality for other devalued groups,
such as girls and women, members of racialized groups,
people with disabilities, people considered overweight, homosexuals, and bisexuals. As a consequence, having mis-
treated and oppressed vast numbers of people and then
calling "abnormal" their reactions to that treatment, our
society has seemed to need vast numbers of therapists to
deal with all this apparent abnormality. Today it is possible to find therapists and therapy or self-help groups specializing in a huge number of problems, situations, or
conditions for which therapy is by no means either a reasonable or an effective solution. Therapist Lottie Marcus
has written of the concerns of patients she has seen:

> How many complaints had their origins in malefi-
> cent social and political environments: brutal work-
> ing conditions, poor schools, slum housing, cultural
> isolation, psychological illegitimacy—things we
> couldn't very well treat in our clinic. Official policy
> was to award "courtesy disease labels" for these
> cases—"depression," "melancholia," "suicidal ide-
> ation"—primarily to cover possible legal contingen-
> cies, but also to satisfy the medical workers' craving
> to feel in control. . . . The same thing occurs in pri-
> vate practice. I often see patients with complaints
> whose origins are largely sociogenic: unresponsive
> institutions, alienating work circumstances, occupa-

tional stress, arbitrary job displacements.... Yet many times, I'm required to award "courtesy disease labels" myself, either to enable clients to receive insurance benefits, and get reimbursed, or provide easily decodable data for colleagues ... our lives as professionals sometimes quarantine us from the "contamination" of that larger world where we and our patients ultimately have to cope, as best we can, with the apocryphal issues we face as parents, citizens, teachers, dreamers, and friends.

One might take the view (as I have done elsewhere) that friendship, consciousness-raising groups, and social action might be more appropriate forums for dealing with the effects of oppression and that they could be more helpful than therapy because they lack the stigma of the latter. But the common model of friendship in North America tends to be extremely limited. Consciousness-raising and social action have gone out of style, their substantial benefits almost forgotten. And we are not supposed to ask too much of our friends, not supposed to ask very personal questions, not supposed to disagree with our friends about important issues. Therapists are everywhere. As a result, as theorist Rachel Perkins has pointed out, when a loved one dies, instead of feeling free to mourn fully and deeply with family and friends, we feel we must see a therapist to help us with our mourning. We fear imposing on family and friends, we wonder if we are mourning "too much" or "for too long" and so need a therapist to help us figure out why we feel so sad—as though losing a loved one is not reason enough to feel deeply sad for a long time. Some therapists and groups are only too happy to play into these attitudes. In principle, there needn't be anything wrong with joining a therapy or self-help group. But in reality, the impression that a therapy patient is someone who is sick or broken and in need of fixing, rather than someone who needs understandable human caring and support during a difficult time, has meant that being "in therapy" makes people feel that something is wrong with them. In many self-help groups, rather than the ethos being, "We are here because we can help each other with difficult problems that we share," it is, "We all come from unspeakably horrible backgrounds and screwed-up families, and we are so damaged that we cannot function on our own and need to spend enormous amounts of time sharing our shame and pain." This means that people who are already wrestling with an upsetting situation or feeling now have to do their wrestling under the specter of the belief that they are weird or abnormal as well.

For this reason, Wendy Kaminer's incisive book *I'm Dysfunctional, You're Dysfunctional* struck a powerful chord in many people. With the proliferation of healing and recovery programs for alcohol, drug, and sexual abuse, for "love addiction," for compulsive gambling or use of credit cards, and for a host of other real problems, many people report having been helped in twelve-step groups and similar ones. In more than twenty years as a psychologist, I have learned that no one really knows why some children can live with an emotionally detached father or an alcoholic mother and grow up pretty well and happily but others cannot. Anyone who feels unhappy or scared ought to have the chance to get help in dealing with those feelings, whether through friends, self-help groups, or visits to professional therapists. But what worries me—and what Kaminer describes in telling detail—is that often the professionals make proclamations such as, "Detached fathers destroy their children emotionally," and then everyone who has had a detached father comes to believe they have come from a "dysfunctional" family and are therefore abnormal, sick, and in need of recovery. Let me make it clear that I think that people whose fathers were emotionally detached probably had unhappier times than they would have had if their fathers had been warm and loving, but the nature of human life is that it lacks perfection. Everyone has suffered in some ways. And most people I know find it easier to cope when they do not believe they are emotionally sick. I have frequently been told by patients how vastly different they feel when they think, "I had a detached father, and that has left me with some insecurities or fears or tendencies that I need to monitor and work on," than when they think, "I had a detached father, so my family was dysfunctional, so I am a damaged person." The "mentally ill," "dysfunctional," and "damaged" labels become additional burdens and sources of worry and shame.

In *Psychotherapy: The Purchase of Friendship*, William Schofield says that if we live in an age of anxiety, perhaps it is because we have chosen to be anxious about anxiety. Anxiety, fear, and guilt are—in some measure—unavoidable aspects of human lives. We need to recognize them, understand their sources, and find ways to overcome them, get rid of them, or function in spite of them. But if we assume that our lives should be anxiety-, fear-, and guilt-*free*, we shall always feel that life has treated us worse than everyone else.

Normality and the DSM

A human failing does not become a disease simply because it is extreme.

—Peter Breggin, *Toxic Psychiatry*

With our society's tendency to pathologize most people if not everyone, and the pervasiveness of the same tendency in the mental health professions in general, is there room for normality in the *DSM*?

Psychiatrist Gerald Klerman, long a staunch advocate of the *DSM*, equated "mental disorder" with "abnormality" and referred to patients as "ill" in his chapter on diagnostic classification in *The New Harvard Guide to Psychiatry*. With close to four hundred ways to be abnormal in the *DSM-IV*, the edition of the manual that is in use as I write, it's hard to imagine any pathology-oriented therapist being unable to find some way to label just about anyone as abnormal. Even a brief glance at the *DSM-IV* reveals its potential for wholesale classification of everyone as abnormal. If you are shy, you can be labeled the sort of abnormal called Social Phobia in the *DSM*. If you have been abused or have endured other, terribly upsetting events and are thinking about them a great deal, struggling to come to terms with it all, you may be diagnosed as Obsessive-Compulsive or as having a Generalized Anxiety Disorder. If you are afraid of dogs, you may be classified as having a Phobia. In regard to phobias, the *DSM* authors specify that, to be considered phobic, you are supposed to recognize that your fear is excessive or unreasonable. But in a society that loves dogs, people who fear the animals are made to feel that their fear is excessive and unreasonable. If you have been bitten hard by a dog whom you trusted, what *is* a reasonable degree of fear? Do you want a therapist making that judgment for you? Since some airplanes and trains do crash, when does fear about traveling in them become a phobia? Does it depend on the statistical probability of a crash? Is it reasonable to be very frightened of a crash when the chances are one in one thousand that it will happen? How about one in ten thousand or one in one hundred thousand? If being mangled or killed is a likely outcome in the case of an unlikely crash, just how much fear is appropriate?

Another *DSM* category is Immature Personality Disorder. Nowhere do the authors specify what the criteria for that form of abnormality might be; it is left utterly to the judgment of the examining therapist. There is nothing to keep a woman who wishes not to bear children or a person of either sex who wishes to hitchhike around the world, spend a lot of time alone, or try to write the Great American Novel from being regarded as having Immature Personality Disorders. Kirk and Kutchins note that

> for children who are 'argumentative with adults, frequently lose their temper, swear, and are often angry, resentful, and easily annoyed by others' the current psychiatric nomenclature provides a diagnosis of Oppositional Defiant Disorder. . . . Through these criteria, describing common, everyday behaviors of children, the rhetoric of science transforms them into what are purported to be objective symptoms of mental disorder.

With such categories as Nicotine Dependence included in the manual, millions of people will surely be covered. Come to think of it, though, now that so many people have stopped smoking, does that mean that we have a mentally healthier population than before? Have millions of psychiatrically disordered people, by "butting out," shed their abnormalities? The *DSM-IV* includes Minor Depressive Disorder. Very few people would *not* fit that description, especially since it can be as brief as two weeks and does not have to meet any particular number of criteria. Journalist Erica Goode writes that such labels "suggest that any departure from happiness is abnormal" and "encourages people in the questionable belief that life's difficulties are readily fixed by experts."

So many of the categories of abnormality in the *DSM* include criteria that have to be judged by the examining therapist. To receive the diagnosis of Hypoactive Sexual Desire Disorder, a person of either sex must be judged to have "persistently or recurrently deficient sexual fantasies and desire for sexual activity," and "the judgment . . . is made by the clinician." Based on my own experiences with both friends and colleagues who are psychotherapists, I have to say that I worry about what some of them judge to be normal sexuality—in their patients, themselves, and their sexual partners. Many therapists believe that part of the natural course of treatment includes the patient having sexual fantasies about the therapist. In regard to this I have to ask, in desperation, "Have you *seen* how some therapists treat their patients? Do we want to call it normal and healthy to have intense sexual fantasies about someone who sits behind you, rarely speaks, believes that none of your feelings about him or her are *really* about him or her (that they are actually about your father or mother), and believes that they know far more about you than you do about yourself? Would we want our loved ones to have sexual fantasies about people who treat them like that?" Because Hypoactive Sexual Desire Disorder and so many other diagnoses require what the *DSM* authors call "a clinical judgment" about whether the patient meets the criteria, there is wide scope for diagnosing virtually every one of us as mentally ill.

I gave a lecture some years ago called "Do Mental Health Professionals Think There Is a Normal Woman?" Most women, upon seeing the title, laughed out loud, a laugh of recognition because they were acutely aware of the ways their behavior tends to be considered wrong, no matter what they do. If they are reserved, they are regarded as cold and "castrating"; if they are outgoing and expressive, they are considered overly dramatic, intrusive, pushy, and overwhelming. I pointed out that a look at just two *DSM*-III-R categories showed the difficulty of imagining a woman being normal according to that manual. Self-Defeating Personality Disorder (SDPD) and Premenstrual Dysphoric Disorder (PMDD) are two labels that alone are conceivably applicable to nearly all women. SDPD has been called by its critics "good-wife syndrome," because of such criteria as putting other people's needs ahead of one's own and feeling unappreciated. SDPD has also been described as an accurate summary of the consequences of abuse. Many abused women feel ashamed of themselves and unappreciated (understandably) because of having been abused and having been made to feel that they deserved it or brought it on themselves, and many hope they will be treated better if they put their own needs last and try desperately to please other people. To receive the diagnosis of PMDD, you need to have only one of the following characteristics: "marked" feelings of anxiety, anger, irritability, depression, or emotional lability. You also must have four physical symptoms that are extremely common not only among women just before their menstrual periods begin but among women *and* men at any time. These include bloating, changes in appetite, and sleep disturbances. We might well ask what such physical symptoms are doing in a manual of mental illness. And as usual, it is up to your therapist to decide whether your anxiety is "marked" and you are therefore psychiatrically ill. As a result:

- Women who are irritable or angry may well be diagnosed as premenstrually mentally ill, especially if they are not carrying out their traditionally "feminine" wife-and-mother or other caretaking roles.

- Women who are depressed, withdrawn, or self-effacing may be diagnosed as premenstrually mentally ill.
- Women who are carrying out their traditionally "feminine" wife-and-mother roles are likely to be diagnosed as having Self-Defeating Personality Disorder.
- Both women and men who are victims of severe abuse are in danger of being diagnosed as having Self-Defeating Personality Disorder.

When I combined the vast numbers of women who would qualify for the label "abnormal" in the above ways with the very high frequency with which therapists classify mothers as so inadequate or bad that they cause mental illness in their children, I realized that virtually every woman could fall into one or more of those categories. Then, too, when a woman is menopausal, it is unlikely that therapists will diagnose her as psychiatrically disordered for some reason related to her premenstrual changes, but they may well diagnose her as being disturbed due to menopause.

The misinterpretation of behavior as pathology also results quite often from the labeling of *social* problems as individual psychological problems. For instance, in discussing the issue of mental competency, Robert Pepper-Smith and William Harvey described an impoverished older woman who was declared mentally incompetent because she wanted to return home from the hospital even though she could not afford to hire a helper and without assistance she would be in some danger of falling. Her preference for going home was pathologized rather than, for instance, being regarded as a sign of courage in the face of danger or of her valuing autonomy over dependency and fearfulness. And the problem was described not as our culture's inadequate provision of assistance for people in such situations but as the woman's alleged irrationality.

In the past twenty-five years, the APA has produced four editions of its manual, four rather different ways of defining and classifying "mental disorders," each one involving removing some categories, putting some new ones in, and changing others. Surely the people shoved in and out of these pigeonholes have not themselves changed so vastly and so often. What, then, could explain such major alterations? The *DSM* folks would have us believe that solid scientific research has *revealed* more about the "real" nature of mental disorder and the *DSM* has been modified accordingly. But that is not necessarily the case.

One might say that, to be fair, we have to recognize that mental illness is not like physical illness, because with regard to many physical problems, one either has or does not have them. A person either does or does not have tuberculosis or a broken ankle, but many "mental illnesses" are only exaggerated forms of "normality." One could argue that intense focus, for instance, on a forthcoming presentation at work might be considered a sign of mental illness when it crosses the line and becomes constant preoccupation, to the exclusion of everything else, for weeks ahead. But the danger of the *DSM*—or any classification scheme—is that it is used in a system with so little monitoring of decisions about when the line is crossed, and the *DSM* leaves enormous scope for subjectivity, opinion, judgment, and bias in making those decisions.

These, then, are some of the ways in which everyone within reach of the *DSM* or of traditional mental health practitioners is in real danger of being categorized as abnormal. And again let me stress that pathologizing people on a grand scale is by no means limited to psychiatrists. As I write, the current issue of a publication from the American *Psychological* Association includes, with no questioning or critical analysis, a report of a study based on the *DSM* categories, whose authors claim to have "found" that nearly half of the U.S. population has had a mental illness at some time. The following chapter is the story of the steps that the *DSM* authors take that lead to this state of affairs.

4

How the American Psychiatric Association Decides Who Is Not Normal—Part I

One should be able to choose one's mental constructs intelligently, rejecting those that do not serve one's needs or that lead to social injustice.

Barbara Walker, *The Skeptical Feminist*

If you pictured a group of professional therapists and researchers seeking a way to decide who is normal while doing as little harm as possible, my bet is that what the American Psychiatric Association really does would never enter your mind.* If somehow it did, and if you are anything like me, you would tell yourself you are being paranoid, antiauthoritarian, unjustifiably stuck in a habit of assuming that people with power usually abuse it. In this chapter and the next two I tell the story of how the APA carries out its self-appointed task of separating the normal from the abnormal, and I tell it to you as I learned

*Much of this chapter and the next one was taken from my chapter, "Afterword: A warning" in *The myth of women's masochism* (New York: Signet, 1987) and from my article, "How *do* they decide who is normal? The bizarre, but true tale of the *DSM* process." *Canadian Psychology/Psychologie canadienne* 32 (1991): 162–70.

about it myself.* I confine this chapter to the information that came directly to me because here I simply want to tell the story as I saw it unfold. My being a woman and a psychologist and a feminist no doubt affects my presentation of information about the *DSM*. Although I would never deny my biases or feelings in regard to the *DSM*, I have tried to make them as clear as possible. I have also included as many direct quotations as possible from the relevant players, so that the reader can be assured of seeing many of the players' own words.

Throughout most of the history I am about to relate, I think that my attitude was fairly typical of that of the general public and many mental health professionals; it was one of trust that the *DSM* authors' paramount concern was to produce a classification system based on good science and doing as little harm and as much good as possible to their patients. I had learned over the years to think carefully about both research and treatment, and I certainly knew that many mental health professionals—including me, of course—often make mistakes, fail to think clearly, have their own emotional agendas, and so on; but one could not have accurately described my attitude toward the *DSM* as basically distrustful and antagonistic. In fact, recently I came across some lecture notes I had used in a course on psychological assessment until 1985, in which I praised the nice logic of one part of the *DSM-III*, in which one was shown on a "decision tree" the various possible causes of a child's learning problem. In my notes, I also praised the *DSM-III* authors, whose names I did not even know at the time, for having introduced into the manual the concept of the importance of such factors

*Readers wishing to learn more about the historical and political context of the APA and its *DSM* will find Kirk and Kutchins's book *The Selling of DSM* immensely informative.

as poverty in producing emotional distress (factors that turn out to be considered rarely for diagnosis).

It was a disappointing surprise to me, therefore, and one that I acknowledged only a small step at a time, to discover that a careful and sincere search for either scientific support or even usefulness to therapists wanting to help their patients has played only a minor role in the entire process of constructing the *DSM-III*, *DSM-III-R*, and *DSM-IV*. Many other factors did figure significantly, including APA personnel's worries about what the public and their patients would think of psychiatrists, the force with which they resisted examining their own biases in their clinical practice, and a host of other political and probably financial considerations. Psychiatrist Mark Zimmerman, who assisted with the *DSM-III-R* revisions, urged, "In the 1990s and beyond, changes in psychiatric nosology [that is, classification] should follow science." As you are about to see, changes in the *DSM* do nothing of the kind. In fact, the *DSM* process's major weakness is that mental disorders are defined so much on the basis of the beliefs and values of those who literally write the book. Chapter 7 is a description of the scarcity of good science and the pervasiveness of politics, power, and other inappropriate determinants of the *DSM* authors' decisions.

As I said in Chapter 1, my involvement with the *DSM* executives began in 1985 when I heard that they were planning to include Masochistic Personality Disorder in their next edition. At that point, because I knew that that label had been used unofficially to heap unjustifiable blame on so many people (mostly women and members of racialized and other devalued groups) by claiming that they brought their problems on themselves and enjoyed suffering, I joined with members of the APA's own Committee on Women and some other therapists to oppose the move.

We also opposed two other *DSM* proposals. One was their intention to designate a form of premenstrual syndrome (PMS) a mental illness, which they first labeled Premenstrual Dysphoric Disorder (PDD). The other was their creation of a category they introduced under the title Paraphilic Rapism (PR). Every category in the manual has both a label and a list of criteria that the person is supposed to meet in order to be given the label. For Paraphilic Rapism, the individual had to have attempted or fantasized about rape and to have experienced intense sexual arousal or desire associated with it for at least six months. A rapist's tendency to think a lot about rape would be used in court by defense lawyers to argue that rapists should go not to prison but instead into psychiatric treatment. It was clear that the diagnosis would be used in this way because that had already happened even though the category was not yet listed in the *DSM*; therapists hired by the defense would interview rapists and testify that the fellows couldn't help themselves and, in essence, weren't evil but just emotionally disturbed and therefore ought not to go to jail but needed therapy. This claim was frequently made despite the fact that therapy had not been shown to stop rapists from raping again. In a similar way, women who had been battered or raped had long been blamed, both in and out of courtrooms, for bringing the violence on themselves by their allegedly provocative or masochistic behavior, and so their batterers and rapists had been absolved of responsibility through the labeling of the victims as psychologically twisted or mentally ill. The *DSM-III-R* proposal to give Masochistic Personality Disorder official status in the handbook would have increased the apparent legitimacy of that category and made it seem like a genuine "mental disorder," too, even though, as I shall describe, there was and is no evidence that such a condition exists. The masochism and rapism categories, taken together, would have meant excusing rapists for their crimes because their own alleged mental disorder (PR) meant they should not be held responsible for their actions, but their *victims* were to have been regarded as causing the rape by *their* alleged mental disorder of masochism, a need to force others to make them suffer. (Table 1 is a description of SDPD as it appeared in the *DSM-III-R*.)

Table 1. Self-Defeating Personality Disorder

A. A pervasive pattern of self-defeating behavior, beginning by early adulthood and present in a variety of contexts. The person may often avoid or undermine pleasurable experiences, be drawn to situations or relationships in which he or she will suffer, and prevent others from helping him or her, as indicated by at least five of the following:

1. chooses people and situations that lead to disappointment, failure, or mistreatment even when better options are clearly available
2. rejects or renders ineffective the attempts of others to help him or her
3. following positive personal events (e.g., new achievement), responds with depression, guilt, or a behavior that produces pain (e.g., an accident)
4. incites angry or rejecting responses from others and then feels hurt, defeated, or humiliated (e.g., makes fun of spouse in public, provoking an angry retort, then feels devastated)
5. rejects opportunities for pleasure, or is reluctant to acknowledge enjoying himself or herself (despite having adequate social skills and the capacity for pleasure)
6. fails to accomplish tasks crucial to his or her personal objectives despite demonstrated ability to do so, e.g., helps fellow students write papers, but is unable to write his or her own

7. is uninterested in or rejects people who consistently treat him or her well, e.g., is unattracted to caring sexual partners

8. engages in excessive self-sacrifice that is unsolicited by the intended recipients of the sacrifice

B. The behaviors in A do not occur exclusively in response to, or in anticipation of, being physically, sexually, or psychologically abused.

C. The behaviors in A do not occur only when the person is depressed.

Note: For coding purposes, record: 301.90 Personality Disorder NOS (Self-Defeating Personality Disorder).

Naive though I may have been, when I heard about the APA's proposals in 1985, I believed that they had somehow failed to understand the dangers inherent in these categories. Once those dangers were pointed out to them, I thought, they would surely change their plans to include them in the *DSM*'s next edition. The APA's Legislative Assembly had responded to the initial protest about their proposals by setting up an Ad Hoc Committee. That committee had met with opponents of the proposals in New York in mid-November and was scheduled to meet with members of the APA's Committee on Women in Washington, D.C., in December 1985, at a time when I was due to be there on other business. The assembly had also suggested that for the meetings, Spitzer's Work Group on Personality Disorders invite representatives both from the American Psychiatric Association's own Committee on Women and from the American *Psychological* Association's Committee for Women in Psychology. The Committee on Women invited me to address the Ad Hoc Committee at its Washington meeting, and that was where I began to learn that it would take more than pointing out the dangers to persuade the APA to change its course. I also began to learn there that respect for scientific procedures is often missing from *DSM* proceedings.

The APA's *DSM-III-R* Task Force was headed by New York psychiatrist Robert Spitzer. Under Spitzer were various work groups for largish classes of diagnostic categories, the relevant one for this chapter being the Personality Disorders Work Group, which Spitzer also headed. For the tremendously important family of diagnoses called personality disorders, then, Spitzer the work group leader answered directly to Spitzer the task force head. Personality disorders are of particular significance because, unlike some other mental disorders, these are defined as maladaptive organizations of the entire personality. (A person who has a fear of heights and a person whose primary source of anguish is shame about sexuality are said to have problems limited to particular aspects of their lives, not to have personality disorders.) Furthermore, historically, personality disorders have been considered extremely difficult, if not impossible, to change, so there is often a sense of throwing up one's hands in helplessness when one confronts an individual who is believed to have a personality disorder.

At November's Ad Hoc Committee meeting, according to psychologist Lenore Walker, a statement by forensic psychologist Lynne Rosewater in the New York meeting stopped the momentum to include the three new diagnoses. Rosewater, then chair of the Feminist Therapy Institute, said that her institute's steering committee "had voted to invest all its financial and other resources in filing a lawsuit" if the APA approved the proposed categories. Rosewater had pointed out that each criterion Spitzer's group had proposed for Masochistic Personality Disorder was behavior that is typical of victims of violence, and so she asserted that "using such a diagnosis . . . [could] violate the civil rights of women by causing irreparable injury and undue hardship to women and victims of violence (most of whom are women)." Also at the New York meeting, Walker had used information from her own research and clinical experience to show how SDPD would further victimize victims.

According to *Time* magazine, at least one psychologist at the November hearings was distressed by the poor quality of thinking displayed by the *DSM-III-R* work group:

> To psychologist Renee Garfinkel, a staff member of the American Psychological Association, "The low level of intellectual effort was shocking. Diagnoses were developed by majority vote on the level we would use to choose a restaurant. You feel like Italian, I feel like Chinese, so let's go to a cafeteria. Then it's typed into the computer. It may reflect on our naivete, but it was our belief that there would be an attempt to look at things scientifically."

In the same *Time* article the following appeared: "Spitzer and his colleagues were happy enough to give up the word *masochism*, but seemed stunned by the determination to chip away at the concept behind it. The feminists seemed surprised and indignant that the meeting descended into the usual picturesque result of successful lobbying: a bit of old-fashioned horse trading." In response to this, Spitzer replied in a December letter to the *Time* editor, "We are scientists and not horse traders." I was to learn in the next eight years that such Nixon-like claims about the righteousness and scrupulousness of the *DSM* committee's procedures—unjustified as they were by the committee's actual conduct—were common practice for the APA and its various bodies.

Lynne Rosewater reported that, during the hearings, "[T]hey were having a discussion for a criterion [about Masochistic Personality Disorder] and Bob Spitzer's wife [a social worker and the only woman on Spitzer's side at that meeting] says, 'I do that sometimes' and he says, 'Okay, take it out.' You watch this and you say, 'Wait a second, *we* don't have a right to criticize *them* because this is 'science'?"

After the November hearings, the *DSM-III-R* authors made a few changes, some of which sounded pretty good but none of which substantially reduced the dangers the SDPD category created. Indeed, the changes may have done actual harm by slightly masking the dangers. The label was changed from Masochistic Personality Disorder to Self-Defeating Personality Disorder (SDPD). The term *masochist* had been associated with Freudian theory, and the work group hoped to appeal to non-Freudians by changing the label, ostensibly to show that one need not believe in a particular theory about how people got that way in order to be able to label their behavior. However, "self-defeating" embodies the same victim-blaming, she-brought-it-on-herself attitude as does "masochistic."

Label-changing is a frequent feature of *DSM* procedures. After the December hearings, the work group changed the Paraphilic Rapism label to Paraphilic Coercive Disorder, a move that made the category's nature and its potential for abuse less obvious. And after the APA's June 28, 1986, Board meeting, Premenstrual Dysphoric Disorder was changed to Periluteal Phase Dysphoric Disorder, a fancy way of saying that sometime around the days just before menstruation begins, women feel bad. This label was again changed by the time of the *DSM-III-R*'s publication to the deceptively scientific-sounding Late Luteal Phase Dysphoric Disorder (LLPDD) (and in

DSM-IV is back to Premenstrual Dysphoric Disorder). The double-barreled power of the LLPDD label was that in two ways it made it harder to criticize, because it made it harder even for most therapists—not to mention the public—to understand. In the first place, few people would readily recognize that Late Luteal Phase Dysphoric Disorder was a fancy name for PMS, making it likely that few would ever even wonder whether this new category needed thoughtful examination. In the second place, the new label gave the impression of great scientific precision, since it seemed that one was no longer dealing with some vague, general time before menstrual bleeding began but rather with some apparently highly specific, clearly identifiable few days in the *late* part of the *luteal* phase of the cycle.

The APA Ad Hoc Committee on *DSM-III-R*'s second set of hearings was convened on December 4, 1985, at APA headquarters in Washington, D.C., with the APA Board of Trustees' next meeting to follow on December 7. The Ad Hoc Committee, chaired by psychiatrist Robert Pasnau, heard presentations in support of the proposed diagnoses from the Work Group to Revise *DSM-III* (chaired by Spitzer) and against the proposals from the APA's Committee on Women and its consultants.

I was present for only the portion of the hearings related to SDPD, but of particular concern to me, as to Garfinkel in November, was the generally poor quality of thinking reflected in the comments and questions of those supporting the diagnoses. One woman psychiatrist supported SDPD on the grounds that she often participates in Catholic annulment proceedings where she is asked to assign diagnoses to the wife and the husband, and she frequently uses "masochistic." I had hoped that such eighteenth-century rationalizations as "Whatever is, is right" had fallen into disuse by now. And a male psychiatrist at the hearings said similarly that this diagnosis had to be adopted because "We see people like this all the time." No, we don't, I explained—we *think* we see people like this; but in fact we are seeing people (usually women) who have very low self-esteem. I pointed out that many therapists had told me that the problem most common to psychotherapy patients *is* poor self-esteem and that, because of this, they had for decades bemoaned the absence of "poor self-esteem" from lists of official psychiatric categories. I suggested that "poor self-esteem" would be far more useful and would indicate a clearer, more productive path for work in therapy than would Self-Defeating Personality Disorder, but they made no response to this suggestion, perhaps because "poor self-esteem" lacks the mystique of jargon and doesn't really sound all that abnormal.

Spitzer asked to respond to my presentation, in which I had briefly stated the reasons that I did not believe people enjoyed suffering or brought defeat on themselves because they enjoyed it. Spitzer began by saying that he had seen me on the "Donahue" show the previous morning (when I had talked about *The Myth of Women's Masochism* and the proposed diagnoses) and that he agreed with almost everything I had said. Of course, if he really had agreed, he would have withdrawn the category from consideration.

The only thoughtful comment came from a man who asked whether we were saying that our society *trains* females to be self-denying and self-effacing and that now the APA wants to label that behavior pathological. That was precisely what we were saying, we assured him, and I went on to point out that no parallel label had been proposed for the *DSM-III-R* for men; that is, no suggestion had been made by the APA that traditionally "masculine" behavior ought to be called pathological. One of the psychiatrists asked me what such a category might be. Looking at the mostly male Ad Hoc Committee and work group, I replied that it might include, for example, a severe difficulty in the ability to express a range of feelings. In response, I was told that the *DSM-III* already had a category for that, Obsessive-Compulsive Personality Disorder, and I replied that that was really not the same thing. The subject was then dropped.

Also at the December hearings, Spitzer expressed dismay about the *Time* magazine article in which Lenore Walker had described what the reporter had called the "horse trading" that went on at the November meetings. Spitzer said that reading Walker's remarks had upset some of his women patients, and Walker replied that she felt it was good for women to read such things.

After feminist psychiatrist Judith Herman summarized the objections of the APA Committee on Women to SDPD, Ad Hoc Committee chair Robert Pasnau suggested that "we adjourn to the—dare I say it—Freud room" to discuss what had just been heard. Those adjourning to the Freud room to decide whether to withdraw or proceed with the SDPD category were members of the Ad Hoc Committee and members of Spitzer's work group; only those of us who opposed the category were excluded. Not surprisingly, the Freud-room group decided not to withdraw the diagnosis. Furthermore, none of the Ad Hoc Committee's recommendations about the proposed categories was made known to the Committee on Women until thirty minutes before they came up on the Board of Trustees' agenda on December 7. This withholding of crucial information from potential opponents until the last possible moment turned out to be a tactic that work groups for both the *DSM-III-R* and the *DSM-IV* would use with great regularity and effectiveness to render the opposition impotent.

By February 1986, the APA's important Joint Reference Committee had recommended that no "controversial" categories be added to the *DSM-III-R*—with no mention of concern about the damage the proposed categories would do to patients, only apparent concerns to protect psychiatrists from further negative publicity and to minimize dissension within the APA.

Opponents of the category, however, did not relax. In March, the strongly feminist Association for Women in Psychology (AWP) met in Oakland and discussed the dangers in the imminent *DSM-III-R*. In the Feminist Therapy Institute's suite there, the plan was conceived to have a demonstration and speak-out at the APA convention in May, and attendees of the AWP business meeting voted to join in a new "Coalition Against Ms . . . Diagnosis." The coalition included representatives from the Feminist Therapy Institute, the Battered Women group, American Psychological Association, American Psychiatric Association, National Association of Women and the Law, and the National Association of Social Workers. Realizing how strong was the opposition to the proposed categories, I drafted a petition on which signers could declare their protest against all three categories (Paraphilic Coercive Disorder, Premenstrual Dysphoric Disorder, and Self-Defeating Personality Disorder), and I gathered signatures there and everywhere else I lectured or went during the next two months. The rapidity with which women of all kinds and many men grasped the destructive potential of the categories was exciting. From audiences of a vast variety, 80 to 90 percent of listeners signed the petitions. The aim was to demonstrate to the APA that their proposed diagnoses were indeed "controversial," that even an unorganized, spontaneous petition campaign had spread like wildfire and the plan for the speak-out had generated enormous enthusiasm, because the dangers were so serious.

As a high school debater, I had learned a healthy respect for the importance of investigating what were often two or more legitimate positions on any issue. But as my colleagues and I have looked, since 1985, for worthy points made by supporters of SDPD and LLPDD, assuming that we might need to modify our positions and searching for common ground between the *DSM* authors and ourselves, we have found nothing above the level of, "We think we see it, so it must be there." This has repeatedly put us in a position like that of the child in the fairy tale who, unlike the majority, would say that the emperor wore no clothes. The absence of compelling arguments from the other side made it extremely easy for us to gather petitions with individual signatures and letters from individuals and groups of various sizes, stating their opposition to the proposed diagnoses and expressing their concern about the dangers they embodied. In fact, the petitions and letters represented more than six million people, mostly from the United States and Canada. The numbers were swelled significantly by the opposition of such massive organizations as the American Psychological Association, the American Orthopsychiatric Association (a large organization composed of mental health professionals of all kinds, teachers, nurses, and nonpsychiatric physicians), the Canadian Psychological Association, the National Organization for Women, and Canada's National Action Committee on the Status of Women. People of both sexes and from all walks of life sent letters and signed petitions in huge numbers. Media coverage was abundant, though often wildly off the mark about the issues.

Support for opposition to the diagnoses came from powerful groups who recognized the dangers. Psychologist Elaine Carmen reported in November 1985 that "the Surgeon General has just convened an extraordinary interdisciplinary group of researchers, clinicians, and service providers with expertise in violence and victims were invited. . . . There was considerable discussion about the proposed diagnosis of masochism," and according to Carmen, that workshop's Working Group on Spouse Abuse— Evaluation and Treatment of Victims condemned the Masochistic Personality Disorder label as "victim-blaming, pejorative, and sexist." In January 1986 the Institute for Research on Women's Health issued a statement of protest against all three proposed diagnoses, and the same month Lenore Walker's report in opposition to the masochism/self-defeating category appeared in the Feminist Therapy Institute's publication *FTI Interchange*. On February 2, 1986, the American Psychological Association's Council of Representatives unanimously passed the following statement:

> The American Psychological Association commends the work of the Committee on Women of the American Psychiatric Association in the revision of DSM-III and supports their efforts to adhere to the scientific standards enunciated in the Council of Representatives August 1985 meeting, as follows:
> . . . The APA adopts the policy that useful diagnostic nomenclature must be (a) supported by empirical data, (b) based on broadly representative data, and (c) carefully analyzed.

Of course, none of the three proposed diagnoses fulfilled any of those three criteria.

On March 29, 1986, Dr. Claire M. Fagin, president of the American Orthopsychiatric Association, sent a letter of protest to Spitzer on behalf of her association's board of directors, expressing their objections to all three diagnoses. And the Spring 1986 *Study Group on Women's Issues Newsletter* of the American Orthopsychiatric Association included a lengthy statement of detailed objections to all three proposed categories.

On May 8 a little-publicized meeting of the American Psychiatric Association's Ad Hoc Committee on the *DSM* was held, perhaps in anticipation of the May 12 speak-out, but no information about the nature or outcome of that meeting was made available to anyone opposing the proposed revisions.

On the morning of May 12 in Washington, D.C., as the American Psychiatric Association's annual convention began, attendees were met by a protest march organized by a collective of women mental health professionals. The collective had planned for the protest to include a speak-out and press conference and, at the request of outgoing APA president Carol Nadelson, had scheduled it for 10:30 A.M. to avoid a time conflict with Nadelson's presidential address. At 10:30, however, Walker learned that an official APA press conference with Spitzer had now been scheduled for 10:30 and was being arranged by the APA's press room staff. Walker went ahead and opened the speak-out, and as it began I headed for Spitzer's conference, where I planned simply to hear what announcements he might make and relay them back to the speak-out, at which I had been scheduled to speak briefly. However, APA press room chief John Blamphin announced as I entered the room that the conference would begin with a ten-minute statement by Spitzer, followed—to my astonishment—by a ten-minute statement by me. As Spitzer talked, the speak-out—which was covered in national media—ended, and the women from the speak-out entered the official press conference, where statements were made by feminist psychiatrists Jean Baker Miller, Marjorie Braude, and Association for Women in Psychiatry head Alexandra Symonds, as well as by me.

At that press conference, proponents of the proposed diagnoses had yet another chance to put forth substantive arguments but once again failed to do so. In response to an expression of concern about the fact that a large proportion of APA members who spoke with us seemed unaware of the proposed diagnoses or controversies about them, Spitzer said that the people making the decisions (the work group, the Ad Hoc Committee, the Board of Trustees) needed to be the ones who were familiar with, and able to evaluate, the relevant research. When a reporter, saying she was "from a major women's magazine," asked him whether the premenstrual disorder was going in the *DSM* because psychiatrists had some treatment to offer beyond the suggestions about vitamins, nutrition, and exercise that her readers could find in popular magazines for women, Spitzer replied that they did not. However, he said, that is the very reason we need to put the category in the *DSM*, because that will make it possible to conduct research to find out what will help. As a longtime researcher, I knew that it was patently untrue that research cannot be conducted on a problem unless it appears in the *DSM*. In fact, the vast majority of research in psychiatry—as well as in psychology, social work, and nursing—is not based on *DSM* categories' criteria.

The day after the press conference, May 13, an official APA symposium-debate was held, organized and chaired by Spitzer. "Pro" and "con" arguments were scheduled for LLPDD and SDPD, but Spitzer chose not to schedule any public debate on Paraphilic Coercive Disorder. Four respected "premenstrual syndrome" researchers were to debate PMDD, Jean Hamilton and Sheryle Alagna (now Sheryle Gallant) against including the category and Sally Severino and Barbara Parry in favor of including it. Jean Baker Miller and I were invited to oppose SDPD and Frederic Kass and Richard Simons to support it.

As I entered the ballroom where the debate was to be held, I met Fred Kass for the first time. Noticing his nametag, I introduced myself. Knowing, I suppose, that I had appeared on "Donahue" and apparently wanting to demean that somehow, Kass's first words to me were, "Donahue hit someone!" (referring to a recent media story that Phil Donahue had hit someone who had insulted his wife). I was rather perplexed by this remark and simply said I was looking forward to the debate. In reply, Kass looked around the room and said to me, "I sure hope my patients don't hear what I'm about to say in this debate." "Why, Fred," I told him, "you shouldn't tell me that. I'll use it against you."

When the debate began, Hamilton and Alagna spoke so eloquently about PMDD that Spitzer told the audience candidly that, had he been a debate judge, he would have declared them the winners. However, by that point it was no surprise that compelling, articulate arguments could not change the minds of those who were intent on getting the diagnosis into the manual.

In the debate about SDPD, Jean Baker Miller focused on the problems in every one of the criteria for the category (see Table 1). Taking a fascinating tack, Miller explained that many of her patients who are the wives of successful men (including psychiatrists), as well as the men themselves, could easily be assigned this label. For example, in regard to Criterion 1, she noted that our society teaches women that becoming a doctor's wife is a pinnacle of achievement; thus, psychiatrists' wives might well have felt when they married that they had made the best possible marital choice. When many such women now find that their husbands are rarely home and are minimally involved with the family, asked Miller, are we now to consider the women self-defeating? Further, Miller noted, those husbands—who in choosing to become hardworking psychiatrists were clearly selecting highly desirable, high-status alternatives—could also be considered "self-defeating" because their involvement in work and their uninvolvement in the richness of family life could be regarded as undesirable alternatives. She made similar comments about the other SDPD criteria.

Miller also discussed the danger that psychiatrists would fail to ask their patients whether they had ever been abused. This was crucial because the criteria for SDPD are so typical of most people's response to being abused that it therefore should surely not be considered a mental disorder, any more than having nightmares after a tour of duty in Vietnam or after having been tortured should be considered pathological.

In my turn, I began by pointing out that Spitzer and his group had spent many months presenting their arguments through numerous official APA publications, but that Dr. Miller and I had been given a total of sixteen minutes in this debate to present other perspectives and information. I then hastily summarized the respects in which SDPD failed miserably to meet the standards of the *DSM* as described by Spitzer himself in the introduction to the manual, and then I had time to present three of the major dangers. In the *DSM-III* introduction, all diagnostic categories within were claimed to have met three standards: to be solidly based in good research, to minimize the amount of subjectivity that can come into play when a therapist is making a diagnosis, and to be atheoretical, based on no particular theory about their causes. Showing that SDPD did not meet the requirement of being based on good research was a breeze, because SDPD's inventors and advocates had only provided one research study—perhaps not surprisingly coauthored by Spitzer himself—in support of their category. That study was so deeply and variously flawed that I had prepared and handed out to the audience a summary called "Nine Problems in the Latest Attempt to Research So-called 'Masochistic Personality Disorder.' " I said,

> In this article, the only thing that the authors 'prove' is that 'masochistic personality' is applied consistently by a few Columbia University Psychiatry Department staff and residents (most or all of whom may have known that one of the authors was spearheading the revisions of *DSM-III* and perhaps that he was proposing 'masochistic personality disorder' as a new category) to a cluster of traits which come from very old clinical—and no research—literature.

I told the audience that I taught an undergraduate course in which our primary aim was to teach students how to evaluate research. I said that each year for the examination we made up a pretend scholarly journal article in which we included every methodological error we could think of, to see if the students could identify them. I said to the audience, "This year we aren't going to have to make one up, because we can use the Kass, McKinnon, and Spitzer article." Also in discussing the poor research base, I cited Spitzer's comment from the press conference the previous day about the need for the decision makers

in APA to be familiar with, and able to evaluate, the research, and I suggested that this was a curious comment,
coming as it did from one of the authors of the methodologically unsound published research paper. Next, I mentioned the one piece of research the SDPD advocates had
recently begun, which involved sending a questionnaire to
some APA members, asking them only to give their opinions about the proposed SDPD *if* they agreed that it
should go in the *DSM*. This kind of method could have
come straight from a textbook on "How to Do Bad Research." Author Louise Armstrong has called this study
"the first attempt in the annals of science to validate a
diagnosis, to establish the existence of a disease/disorder,
by the Peter Pan method: Clap if you believe in fairies."
I was fascinated to find that in the introduction to *DSM-
III-R*, Spitzer reported that "the diagnostic criteria for
Self-Defeating Personality Disorder" were studied by examining the "data" from that questionnaire that was, he
wrote, "distributed to several thousand members" of the
APA (p. xxii). By thus reporting only partial information
about that opinion survey, Spitzer gave the impression that
massive scientific research supported SDPD and did not
report its devastating methodological flaws.

The second standard all *DSM-III* categories were said
to meet was to minimize subjectivity. With respect to
SDPD, I pointed out, there was enormous scope for subjectivity in judging whether or not a person fit every one
of the criteria listed. For instance, how is one to decide
whether or not an individual makes undesirable choices
when better options are available? How is one to decide
whether a person feels unappreciated because that is true
or because they "need" to feel unappreciated? And as Jean
Baker Miller trenchantly asked, do we want to consider
women who have married psychiatrists who are consumed

by their work to be women who have made highly desirable or undesirable choices?

The third major *DSM-III* standard was supposed to be that all categories were atheoretical, that they did not depend on a therapist's believing in or invoking any particular psychological theory. However, to call "self-defeating" a person who is in an unhappy relationship or an unrewarding job is clearly to make a major theoretical assumption: One assumes that the unhappiness is caused by the person's need to be self-defeating, rather than, say, because the partner in the relationship or the boss at work is either distant and unsupportive or actively cruel. To make assumptions about the cause of behavior or feelings is to use theoretical explanations. Thus, a person goes to see a therapist and says, "I am feeling miserable in my marriage," and the therapist gives that person the "self-defeating" label, which necessitates that therapist making the assumption that the person's motivations are self-harmful. In addition, unless other therapists or misguided friends have told the patients they are bringing their problems on themselves, few people will come seeking help, saying, "I am self-defeating." To make such an interpretation, then, the therapist must assume that the self-defeating motivation is unconscious; the therapist has to make inferences about the motives behind the patient's behavior, and the moment one makes an inference, one abandons an atheoretical stance.

To call people self-defeating for behaving in self-denying, self-effacing ways in order to *avoid* punishment and rejection—and in order to receive approval and love—is to insist that their behavior be regarded as pathological whether or not they follow the socially prescribed route. It is relevant to note here that Spitzer wrote in the *DSM-III* introduction that in *DSM-III* "there is an inference that there is a behavioral, psychological, or biological dysfunction [in the disorders in the manual], and that the disturbance is not only in the relationship between the individual and society." Furthermore as the APA's own Committee on Women noted in a report: "The criteria and the diagnosis are an additional burden on women and minority groups where racial and gender stereotypes involve socially reinforced behaviors such as self sacrifice, submission, deferring one's own needs and interests, patience and constancy which are positive traits in traditional roles but are labelled pathology under these criteria."

I noted the danger that SDPD involves of pathologizing victims of abuse by calling their understandable, common reactions to abuse a mental disorder. The more one is abused, the more likely one is to feel unappreciated, to put other people's needs ahead of one's own in the hope of avoiding abuse, and so on, and these are SDPD criteria. In fact, to respond any other way to being seriously abused would be rather amazing and is rather rare. But since it is still fairly unusual for many therapists to inquire about histories of abuse, and even when they inquire, patients are often reluctant to talk about it in early sessions, the source of the behavior that becomes labeled as self-defeating is completely missed. Rosewater refers to the sample studied for the originally proposed Masochistic Personality Disorder. In this study, which involved 367 patients, with an average time in treatment of sixteen months, the mental health practitioners who worked closest with these clients were unaware how many were current victims of violence. Related to this problem is that many people who are depressed show the kinds of behavior listed under SDPD. SDPD constitutes a real danger of distracting therapists from a person's depression because this other, albeit mistaken and invalid, label is readily available. And to miss depression in a person is extremely serious, because with depression can come the risk of suicide.

In their part of our debate, Kass and Simons, pushing for the diagnosis, failed to present substantive arguments. Simons, president of the American Psychoanalytic Association, praised my book and then said that he had used it as the basis for a formulation he would then present on a slide. His slide illustrated, he said, that nurturance and altruism were healthy forms of behavior, that "sexual masochism" was a severe disorder and belonged at the opposite end of the continuum, and that in between was "self-defeating" behavior. Implicitly appealing to us to trust therapists who would use the *DSM-III-R*, he assured us that only people displaying "self-defeating behavior" would be diagnosed as having SDPD. In my response I pointed out that having a continuum on a slide does nothing at all to reduce the subjectivity of the therapist who decides whether a particular person's behavior is "self-defeating." I closed by making two final points: (1) I said that nearly every major public supporter of this diagnosis had told me privately that he agreed with everything I wrote in my book, and since what I wrote constituted a series of arguments against SDPD as a diagnosis, I wondered how they managed to reconcile their agreement with my arguments and their support of the diagnosis. I wondered further why they did not publicly acknowledge that agreement. (2) I presented the signatures that had been collected on our petitions and listed just some of the names of organizations that had written to the APA to protest the diagnoses. I reminded the audience that a major APA committee called the Joint Reference Committee and—I had been informed—its Assembly had gone on record as opposing the adoption of any "controversial" diagnoses. In view of the petitions and the letters of protest, I asked, "How controversial is it going to have to get?"

In the discussion period following the debate, psychiatrist Judith Herman asked the pointed question that, in view of what the audience had just heard about the multitude of problems involved in the diagnoses, "What is the rush to get them into *DSM-III-R*?" Treating this question as though it were rhetorical, Spitzer moved to close the debate, but Herman repeated the question and requested an answer. Simons offered to respond and claimed that the "reason" was that these diagnoses were "long overdue" and should have gone into the previous edition.

Two points became crystal clear during the 1985–86 events. One was that the proponents of the new categories felt no obligation to meet the standards that had been claimed for categories in the previous edition of the manual; that is, the categories were not based solidly on good research, were not atheoretical, and were not designed to minimize the need for subjective judgments by therapists. The other was that, in the face of powerful, substantive arguments, only arrogance and insensitivity could have allowed these people to push ahead as far and as hard as they did.

Just before the APA Board of Trustees' late June 1986 meeting, I sent a letter to all members of the Board, summarizing the concerns about the diagnoses' failure to meet the manual's own standards and informing them that I had sent to their new president, Robert Pasnau, copies of the petitions and letters of protest that we had collected. I also informed them that millions of people were represented by the protest. Shortly before the Board voted on the proposed diagnoses, speeches were made to the Ad Hoc Committee and to the Board by various people, including—according to Teresa Bernardez—objections to the proposals from both of the women Board members, Carol Nadelson and Elissa Benedek. Bernardez also reported that Pasnau discussed with the Board the importance of both the scientific validity concerns and the social and political issues involved, indicating the magnitude of the protest.

Amazingly, on June 28, the Board voted 10 to 4 (according to Bernardez) to defeat the proposals. Specifically, what they did was to discard altogether the Paraphilic Coercive Disorder and to vote to create a *DSM-III-R* appendix for "provisional categories needing further study" and to include in it the diagnoses of SDPD and PMDD. As noted earlier, at this time they changed the title of Premenstrual Dysphoric Disorder to Periluteal Phase Dysphoric Disorder. We assumed that the categories in the appendix could not be considered formal, legitimate diagnoses, in view of the way the appendix was to be described. This seemed to be a stunning victory. The only better step they could have taken would have been to discard all three categories entirely; such bodies tend to be loath to take such a step because it alienates their colleagues on such committees as the work group and because it calls into question their credibility as an association, since the APA Board had had chances to defeat the proposals several times before but had nevertheless charged right ahead. As one senior APA official told me privately, Board members who leaned toward discarding all three categories were accused by their colleagues of "giving in to the women," a comment frighteningly reminiscent of little boys' taunt, "You don't wanna play with the girls!"—hardly solid grounds for making decisions.

Believing that something good had been achieved, however, would have been premature. Spitzer claimed that some Board members favoring the appendix disagreed about what placing categories in an appendix should mean, and he proposed what he called, incredibly, a "compromise." According to that proposal, each diagnosis in the "provisional" appendix would have an official number, just like each fully approved diagnosis listed in the main part of the text, and psychiatrists would be told to go ahead and use them as though they were official. In December 1986, just before the Board was to make its final decisions, I sent the Board members a letter asking why, when only a single study of "MPD/SDPD" had ever been done, an official APA press release mislabeled the research on the category as "substantial." The Board went ahead and approved both categories for inclusion in the appendix, and the appendix was called "Proposed diagnostic categories needing further study." They were listed with official numbers, there was no warning to clinicians *not* to use the labels until and unless they were validated by future research, and in the years following the 1987 publication of *DSM-III-R*, the allegedly provisional categories were widely used without much regard for their unproven, unsupported status.

When the *DSM-III-R* was published, the fact that the task force had baldly lied became clear. Although SDPD and LLPDD were included in the provisional appendix, LLPDD was also listed in the main text of the manual, which is supposedly reserved for fully tested and scientifically supported diagnoses. To list a category and its criteria in a provisional appendix, with the category label alone in the main text, had never been done before and is hard to explain: If the category was valid, couldn't it be fully described in the main text? And if it was not valid, shouldn't it be kept out of the main text? Perhaps the difficulty of explaining the split led to the false claim that LLPDD was only in the provisional appendix.

Spitzer was to repeat the identical lie some seven years later in regard to the manual's subsequent edition, *DSM-IV*. Furthermore, the pro-*DSM* authors in the 1988 book *The New Harvard Guide to Psychiatry* discussed SDPD "without mentioning the controversy surrounding it, the threatening implications for women, or any relationship between the diagnosis and a history of childhood abuse."

The events just described are cast in a useful perspective when we realize that fewer than two hundred people are listed as having been consulted in the production of the *DSM-III-R*—mostly psychiatrists, males, and whites—a small and limited group to have so much power to make pronouncements about normality and mental health and disorder. Their power to define "truth" is reflected in the fact that in the 1988 *New Harvard Guide to Psychiatry*, psychiatrist Gerald Klerman wrote, "[The] judgment [to put SDPD in the appendix] did not involve controversy over the reliability or validity of the syndrome"—a totally unfounded claim.

Onward to *DSM-IV*

Hardly had the *DSM-III-R* been published when work was announced on the next edition of the manual, this time to be headed by another New York–based white male psychiatrist, Allen Frances (who later moved to Duke University). Clearly, a major issue would be whether to throw out SDPD and LLPDD, confine them to the provisional appendix, or list them in the main text, with fully approved status. In theory, those decisions were to be based on the nature of the new research that was expected to appear in the coming years. Maureen Gans, a graduate student who as an undergraduate had been a key worker in the 1985–86 petition and letter-writing campaign, met with me, and we decided to read the new research on the controversial categories as it was published over the next few years and write evaluations of it.

I phoned Allen Frances to tell him of the work that we planned to do and offered to send his task force our bibliographies and critiques. I also said that we wondered if we might be sent the bibliographies and any other materials produced by them as they carried out their mandate. In reply, he invited me to serve as a consultant to the SDPD subcommittee and an advisor to the LLPDD one. (I never did learn what difference there was between a consultant and an advisor or precisely what either one was supposed to do.) I told him that I had actively and publicly protested the inclusion of those categories in the previous edition, but he said that he knew that and wanted me to work with them because he intended to involve people with varying viewpoints. He also said that all decisions for the upcoming edition were going to be based heavily on the empirical support for each diagnosis. I was impressed and thought that that sounded as though their procedures were going to be more open and less riddled with politics and biases than before, and I agreed to serve, taking care to say that I would feel free to comment publicly if I had concerns about what they did. I was even more encouraged to see a memo from Dr. Frances to the members of the *DSM-IV* Work Group, dated September 19, 1988, in which he declared, "Essentially we are undertaking a scientific assessment project. . . . It is essential that our efforts proceed in as systematic and scientifically based a manner as possible."

SDPD: "Let Nature Take Its Course"
On February 27, 1989, I received a telephone call from Susan Fiester, the psychiatrist who was to chair the Self-Defeating Personality Disorder subcommittee, for which

I was to be a consultant. Presumably because we were supposed to work together, she asked whether I had written anything about SDPD, and I replied that my concerns had been detailed in a new chapter called "Afterword: A Warning," in the 1987 paperback edition of my book *The Myth of Women's Masochism*. Strangely, she declined my offer to send her a copy and said she would obtain one herself. She also told me she would send me copies of a number of unpublished sets of data relevant to SDPD, so Maureen Gans and I could include them in our review of post-*DSM-III-R* research.

In May, having heard nothing and received nothing from her, I wrote to jog her memory and to repeat my request that she send us the unpublished work. I informed her that we wanted to work with her subcommittee but were not sure how to proceed without further word from her. I said that Maureen and I had done the preliminary work for our review and found, so far, that there was still very little empirical research about the category and that what research existed was not very well done and certainly did not warrant the inclusion of SDPD in any form in any diagnostic handbook.

At the end of May, we received a few unpublished articles from Fiester; and wrongly assuming they were the only ones she had available to her, we began to write our review. On July 10, Fiester wrote to tell us that she was completing both a bibliography and a review of the research about SDPD. She promised to send us the bibliography "within the next week" and said that when I received it I could write directly to the authors of the unpublished work to request copies of their papers. We never received her bibliography, and she did not send her review until well after the Personality Disorders Work Group (of which her subcommittee was a part) had met and the deadline had passed for getting feedback about her review to her (more about that later). Although a bibliography was appended to her review when we finally received it, nothing she sent provided information about where the authors of the unpublished papers could be reached, and my several subsequent letters of inquiry to Fiester about this went unanswered.

In the same July 10 letter, Fiester assured me of the "importance of examining the empirical data base . . . and using these reviews as a basis for the proposed disposition of the categories" and said that the research would undergo "careful scrutiny." In that letter she also informed me that she had shown her preliminary review to other members of her subcommittee, but we never saw that preliminary one.

Although we had never been told exactly when our own review would have to be finished in order to be useful to the SDPD subcommittee, we completed it as rapidly as possible and sent copies to Frances, Fiester, and John Gunderson, chair of the Personality Disorders Work Group. On October 16, Gunderson—who ranked between Frances and Fiester in the *DSM-IV* hierarchy—wrote to thank us for the copy of our review but informed us: "Unfortunately, it arrived right after our Work Group has met and discussed issues related to its inclusion or exclusion. The outcome of our discussion was that existing evidence is insufficient to move it in either direction." "Move it in either direction" presumably referred to the possibilities of moving SDPD from the provisional appendix into the main body of the book or leaving it out of the manual altogether. Gunderson further wrote, "The ultimate fate of SDPD in DSM-IV will be tied to any new evidence which can tip the present balance." The results of both our review and the review by Judith Herman, a psychiatrist and expert on abuse, make it abundantly clear that the balance of well-done research for and against SDPD is not delicate at all. In fact, there is virtually no scientifically legitimate, empirical evidence to show that there *is* such a thing as SDPD or something like it.

Curiously—in light of Gunderson's claim about the committee's belief that there was insufficient evidence yet to move SDPD either way—Frances wrote on October 26 to say he was "pleased that [SDPD] does not engender enthusiasm in the Personality Disorders Work Group and I feel hopeful that it will not appear at all in DSM-IV." He also thanked me for our review but called some of our article "a bit too polemical" and observed that he didn't "see any need for heated controversy given the current process."

Having thus been urged to have faith in the process but having received apparently contradictory letters from Gunderson and Frances, I wrote to Frances on November 8 about Gunderson's letter saying there was insufficient evidence to move the category either way and his own letter saying that SDPD did not engender enthusiasm in the work group and therefore probably would be left out, but he did not respond. I also wrote to Gunderson:

> I was not surprised by the nature of the decision not to "move it in either direction," although I had previously accepted at face value Dr. Frances' statement to me . . . that any category without a sound empirical basis would be excluded. . . . What kind of "balance" is there in a field in which, as you saw in our review, there is simply not one shred of evidence in support of the category?

As one more addition to the burgeoning complexity of contradictions, the same Gunderson who on October 16 had expressed regret that our review had arrived too late to be considered by the committee then wrote on November 14 that our review "was an important source of material for the discussion we had about the fate of . . . SDPD" at that very same meeting. And in fact, the minutes he sent me of that meeting, although quite long and detailed, include no mention whatsoever of either our review or Herman's review. We only learned that Herman was serving as an advisor or consultant to the SDPD subcommittee and had written a critique of the literature when she sent us her review in December 1989.

On November 17, Fiester sent us her review of the research on SDPD. The Personality Disorders Work Group's minutes from their October meeting had included a reminder that comments on Fiester's review should be forwarded to her by October 24, so I could not have made the deadline. With the review came Fiester's offer to give me the telephone numbers of the authors of the unpublished data to which she referred in her review (but which she never actually provided, despite the repeated requests I then sent) and her promise to call me "to further discuss your views on Self-defeating Personality Disorder and your critique of my review." After that, and to this day, I never heard another word from her.

Although the deadline for getting feedback to Fiester had passed by the time she sent me her critique, I read her paper and wrote comments about it, which I sent on November 28 to her, Gunderson, and Frances. My comments included observations about the inadequacy of her paper, as well as about her pro-SDPD conclusions that were not supported by the very work that she both cited and partially described elsewhere in her paper. For instance, in my critique I noted that she cited, as though it were methodologically sound, a study that has been shown in published work to have nine major methodological errors; that she presented, as though they were comprehensive, only a few of the concerns about SDPD that had been raised by the APA's Committee on Women; and that she made numerous other errors of varying degrees of complexity and subtlety.

When I sent Fiester my critique of her review, I told her:

> I had very little time to write this critique, and so I am afraid I have not soft-pedalled it as much as I might have. I do have to say that I continue to be as profoundly concerned about the push to keep SDPD in the DSM—even after reading your review—as I have been from the beginning. I have great trouble understanding the powerful motives that must be behind this diagnostic category, because—as you no doubt realize from having read the sloppy empirical literature on SDPD yourself— the empirical basis is absolutely lousy. If a Master's or Doctoral student were to use the available empirical literature to justify it, that student would never have had such a proposal accepted either by me or by any of my colleagues. Do you understand the source of this intense energy behind the SDPD?

I was interested to note that Fiester made the important point in her paper that including a clause specifying that the diagnosis should not be given if abuse had caused the symptoms would probably be ineffective because of clinicians' tendency not to ask about abuse and because of patients' tendency to repress their memories of abuse.

Believing that a critique of the SDPD literature needed to be made widely available for scrutiny, Gans and I submitted our review to the *American Journal of Psychiatry* but heard in January 1990 that it had been rejected. Perhaps that is not surprising, since that journal is an official publication of the American Psychiatric Association. After removing every word that we felt might be considered "polemical" or "strident," we then submitted it to the *Journal of Personality Disorders*, which in 1987 had published an article in which I described the state of the empirical basis at that time for SDPD. In April 1990 we were notified that our article had been soundly rejected. We had submitted the article to Dr. Theodore Millon, who was listed as the journal's editor. From the letterhead of the rejection note, we learned that his coeditor was Allen Frances, and members of the editorial board (who might have included the unnamed individuals who reviewed and rejected our submission) included John Gunderson, Susan Fiester, Robert Spitzer, and Spitzer's frequent coauthor, who is also his wife, Janet Williams.

The *JPD* reviewers' comments on our paper included some intriguing remarks. One reviewer announced, "The authors of this manuscript have a bias. They are opposed to SDPD as a psychiatric category." It did not appear to matter that our opposition had grown partly from our discovery of the shoddy empirical basis for the category, which we described in the article. We were not told the reviewers' identities, but this reviewer referred to us as "they," suggesting knowledge that knew there were two of us; so the reviewer did not read our paper "blindly," unaware of the authors' identities, although blind reviews are accepted practice to guard against bias. The same reviewer said that in our paper we "often use affectively toned descriptors to exaggerate their points" and then gave as examples our words, "all of these measures have *highly unsatisfactory* or *nonexistent* data on their reliability and validity" (reviewer's emphasis).

The other reviewer took us to task because

> Robert Spitzer is purported to have stated that the
> DSM categories must be solidly based in good re-
> search, as stated in the introduction to DSM-III and
> DSM-III-R. This is a simplification of a complex
> issue and Spitzer has never asserted that all of the
> DSM categories are based on or can be justified by
> good empirical research.

In fact, Spitzer had written that "DSM-III reflects an increased commitment in our field to reliance on data as the
basis for understanding mental disorders" and also that
the task force members shared a commitment to ensure
in *DSM* "consistency with data from research studies bearing on the validity of diagnostic categories." Furthermore,
it is interesting that the reviewer, whoever it was, felt familiar enough with Spitzer to claim unequivocally that
Spitzer "has never" made a particular assertion. One has
to wonder about the ethics of choosing a reviewer with
such intimate knowledge of Spitzer, a major proponent of
SDPD, to evaluate our paper.

On January 29, 1990, I felt it was time to express the
full range of my concerns about the *DSM* process to Allen
Frances, so I wrote him a lengthy letter in which I summarized much of what I have described above. The major
issues included the lack of scientific integrity and the various problems with communication. On February 7, he
wrote me a brief letter in which he ignored the substantive
points I made and offered instead an unsolicited opinion
about what he believed to be the reason for my concerns:

> I think we differ only in emphasis and sense of ur-
> gency. The Personality Disorders Work Group is

> aware of all the many problems with SDPD. . . . I
> think your disappointment at the pace and intensity
> of our work in this area reflects that it has a much
> higher priority for you. . . . I think we should let
> nature take its course.

I thought it curious, but perhaps not surprising, that he would equate the scandalous *DSM* process with "nature," implying that the *DSM* group's ways were natural and, therefore, right.

The minutes of the March 1990 meeting of the Personality Disorders Work Group contained the following lines, which at first seemed encouraging:

> SDPD—Dr. Frances mentioned that the group should
> be aware of the concerns of colleagues about the status
> of this disorder. A consensus of the group is that there
> is little enthusiasm for elevating SDPD to become an
> official diagnosis due to lack of empirical support.

However, appended to the minutes was a detailed description of changes to be made in specific SDPD criteria. Furthermore, no mention was made of removing it from the appendix or excluding it from the next edition of the manual entirely.

On November 8, 1990, all my hopes for a scientific and fair way of producing the next *DSM* dashed, I wrote to Allen Frances, resigning from my positions on the SDPD and LLPDD groups. I told him that I was disturbed by their process, and I asked that my name be neither listed nor counted in any of their reports about the people with whom they had worked. I wished neither to be associated with the process nor to be used to swell the number of people they would claim to have consulted.

I heard no more about SDPD until 1992, when I was contacted by Dr. Margaret Jensvold, a psychiatrist who had filed a lawsuit against the National Institute of Mental Health (NIMH) because of having been sexually harassed and subjected to sex discrimination while working there. When Jensvold expressed concern about this treatment, her boss, David Rubinow, who was one of those who had discriminated against her, told her that she had to go into psychotherapy if she wanted to succeed at NIMH. He gave her the names of three male psychiatrists, and she went to speak with one of them. After she had seen him several times, she learned that her therapist was salaried by NIMH, and Rubinow was responsible for his annual contract renewals. Understandably, she became deeply concerned about whether or not he would keep confidential the things that she told him, many of which were about their boss. Jensvold reports that she asked him repeatedly whether he could guarantee her confidentiality, and he never would promise that he would. She continued to see him anyway, because she was quite isolated and was hoping to obtain some help and support. When the therapist's files were examined in preparation for the litigation against NIMH, it was found that, when Jensvold had asked him about confidentiality, he had recorded that she was paranoid. Furthermore, he had written in his notes that she suffered from "Self-Defeating Personality Disorder." That would indeed be the perfect defense for people accused of sexual harassment and sex discrimination: It really wasn't our fault or within our control, because the victim has SDPD and therefore brought it on herself. It is a kind of childish but extremely dangerous way of saying, "Her mental disorder made us do it!"

Jensvold's case became public, and she and Ginger Breggin, who was working with her to help publicize this kind of institutional mistreatment, described it as the "Tailhook of the Medical Establishment." As a result, a several-part series about sexism at NIMH appeared on television, coverage appeared in many publications, and the *Journal of the American Medical Association* announced that it planned to have a reporter cover the trial. Jensvold was invited to appear on television's "Donahue" show about victims of sexual harassment. The focus was on the tendency for those who report the harassment to be cast as the villains, either by being accused of being sexual harassers themselves or by being pathologized as Jensvold had been. Shortly before that program was broadcast but after the other publicity described above, we heard from Judith Herman that the Personality Disorders Work Group had suddenly voted to take SDPD out of the manual's next edition (*DSM-IV*). I appeared on the "Donahue" show with Jensvold and with great pleasure announced this decision. The audience applauded the decision, but I pointed out that we ought not to relax about this matter. I explained that, through seven full years of being shown how scientifically insupportable and also how dangerous the category of SDPD was, the work group had not budged. Their dramatic turnaround came at the point when SDPD suddenly received wide, adverse publicity, damaging the APA's credibility. People who make decisions on such grounds obviously do not have their hearts in those decisions. There was no evidence that they withdrew the category because they had realized it was right to do so, and I feared that it would reappear at some later date, perhaps under yet another label.

As the next chapter shows, the events related to the fate of LLPDD in *DSM-IV* were no less disturbing than those related to SDPD.

5

How the American Psychiatric Association Decides Who Is Not Normal—Part II

LLPDD: Do Half a Million American Women Go Crazy Once a Month?

I had been invited to serve on the LLPDD committee by *DSM-IV* head Allen Frances in late 1988, at the same time that he had asked me to serve on the SDPD one. The former committee's mandate was to review the literature about LLPDD and decide whether to continue to list it for *DSM-IV* in the provisional appendix and also in the main text (as it had been in *III-R*), to list it only in the appendix, to list it in the main text only, or to remove it from the manual altogether. From the moment of that invitation until I ended my official involvement with the *DSM* on November 8, 1990, I received only six brief, minimally informative letters from the LLPDD subcommittee chair, Judith Gold. In those letters, Gold, a psychiatrist working in Halifax, Nova Scotia, merely asked me formally to serve as an advisor to her work group; said her group would inspect all of the relevant literature and "come to some conclusion as to what clinical entity, or entities, if any, exist"; promised to look at the various sociocultural and political issues involved; promised to send me her group's literature review (which she never did); said she looked forward to our review and to our comments on theirs; and thanked us for sending her our bibliography. Graduate students Joan McCurdy-Myers and Maureen Gans and I went ahead and studied the research related to LLPDD (see Table 1 for the *DSM* Task Force's description of LLPDD), wrote a review of it, and in March or early April of 1990 sent a copy of our review to Gold, but we never received a reply. As a result, before I resigned from the two *DSM-IV* subcommittees, most of my conversations and correspondence with other *DSM* people were focused on SDPD and DDPD rather than LLPDD.

I resigned in 1990 as a consultant and advisor because of my concern about the *DSM* Task Force's false claims to base their decisions on science and about their distortions and lies. After that, I heard nothing more of LLPDD until February 19, 1993. At that time, I was notified by psychologist Mary Brown Parlee, a longtime researcher in the field of "premenstrual syndrome," that the *DSM* Task Force had decided to keep LLPDD in the manual for the *DSM-IV* edition, even though the research clearly did not justify it. She said that the LLPDD committee had not been able to agree on a recommendation and that two other people had made the final decision about what to recommend. (Months were to pass before we could find out who those two people were.) Parlee informed me that even the studies published since the paper I had written with McCurdy-Myers and Gans failed utterly to support calling any form of "premenstrual syndrome" a mental disorder. She also said that research failed to show that any form of drug treatment—which was what the LLPDD committee was advocating—was useful. We also discussed our concerns about the harm to women that has resulted from claims that their hormonal changes make them mentally disordered. Over the course of the next few weeks, we learned from the *DSM* Task Force's statements to the media that the plan was not only to maintain LLPDD in the provisional appendix but also to list it in the main text under "Depressive Disorders."

Table 1. Late Luteal Phase Dysphoric Disorder (later retitled Premenstrual Dysphoric Disorder)

A. In most menstrual cycles during the past year, symptoms in B occurred during the last week of the luteal phase and remitted within a few days after onset of the follicular phase. In menstruating females, these phases correspond to the week before, and a few days after, the onset of menses. (In nonmenstruating females who have had a hysterectomy, the timing of luteal and follicular phases may require measurement of circulating reproductive hormones.)

B. At least five of the following symptoms have been present for most of the time during each symptomatic late luteal phase, at least one of the symptoms being either (1), (2), (3), or (4):

1. marked affective lability, e.g., feeling suddenly sad, tearful, irritable, or angry
2. persistent and marked anger or irritability
3. marked anxiety, tension, feelings of being "keyed up," or "on edge"
4. markedly depressed mood, feelings of hopelessness, or self-deprecating thoughts
5. decreased interest in usual activities, e.g., work, friends, hobbies
6. easy fatigability or marked lack of energy
7. subjective sense of difficulty in concentrating
8. marked change in appetite, overeating, or specific food cravings
9. hypersomnia or insomnia
10. other physical symptoms, such as breast tenderness or

swelling, headaches, joint or muscle pain, a sensation of "bloating," weight gain

C. The disturbance seriously interferes with work or with usual social activities or relationships with others.

D. The disturbance is not merely an exacerbation of the symptoms of another disorder, such as Major Depression, Panic Disorder, Dysthymia, or a Personality Disorder (although it may be superimposed on any of these disorders.)

E. Criteria A, B, C, and D are confirmed by prospective daily self-ratings during at least two symptomatic cycles. (The diagnosis may be made provisionally prior to this confirmation.)

Note: For coding purposes, record: 300.90 Unspecified Mental Disorder (Late Luteal Phase Dysphoric Disorder).

After Parlee and I spoke that day in February, I composed the following petition and sent it by regular mail and electronic mail to people I thought would be interested, including members of the various media:

URGENT: CAN YOU HELP?
The American Psychiatric Association plans to include Premenstrual Syndrome in its "bible of mental disorders," the Diagnostic and Statistical Manual of Mental Disorders. Whether or not you believe there is such a thing as PMS—women experiencing some mood or behavior changes shortly before menstruation—it should not be classified as a mental illness.

Please read the information below, gather signatures on the attached petition (feel free to make copies for more signatures), tear off the petition page, and mail it to:

Dr. Joseph English, President
American Psychiatric Association
1400 K Street N.W.
Washington, D.C. 20005

The arguments against including "Premenstrual Dysphoric Disorder" in the *DSM* are:

1. *There is NO sound empirical basis for such a category.* Such researchers as Mary Brown Parlee, Anne Fausto-Sterling, Paula Caplan, Joan McCurdy-Myers, and Maureen Gans have documented that enormous numbers of studies have been done, but most are profoundly flawed and certainly do not constitute evidence that there should be such a disorder. Indeed, the DSM –subcommittee studying PMS reached an impasse about whether or not it should go in the handbook and took the curious step of asking two other people to review the research and decide what should be done.

2. *Such a category carries social and political dangers for women.* There is no parallel category for men, no suggestion that well-documented mood and behavior changes that result from variations in "male hormones" should be given the label of mental illness (no "Testosterone-based Aggressive Disorder").

• There is no sex-blind category for reasonably normal mood or behavior changes caused by physiological problems (no "Post-Influenza Depression").

• At Senate confirmation hearings, job interviews, custody proceedings, and mental competence hearings, women could be asked, "Have you been diagnosed as having Premenstrual Dysphoric Disorder?"

Then followed a petition with the words, "We, the undersigned, oppose the inclusion of 'Premenstrual Dysphoric

Disorder' in the *Diagnostic and Statistical Manual of Mental Disorders*."

Signed petitions again began to pour into the APA office, and many copies were sent to me as well. The media began to pick up on the story, and Judith Gold and I were interviewed on CBC radio's national show "As It Happens." After I said that the literature review I had coauthored showed that there is no scientific justification for claiming that a form of PMS is a mental disorder, Gold asserted that new studies proved me wrong. It is always easy to make such an assertion on a brief show, when one is unlikely to be required to document it.

Soon afterward, Gold and I appeared on "Donahue," where I remarked that the proposed category would result in the labeling of at least five hundred thousand women in the United States alone as mentally disordered in this way. Gold claimed that that was not true, that they were only talking about a very small percentage of women. I replied that both of our statements were correct, but that even a small percentage meant a large number and that, *using Gold's LLPDD group's own statistics* from an official APA publication, we had come up with a conservative estimate of half a million women who would receive the LLPDD diagnosis. She again denied it.

To Gold's and my next joint appearance, I came prepared. We were on the national CBC television show "Midday," and when I brought up the five hundred thousand women and Gold predictably denied it, I held up to the camera the APA publication *DSM-IV Update*, in which the pertinent statistics appeared. This is what the *Update* reported: Surveys of 1,089 women had shown that, of women coming to clinics with complaints that they described as premenstrually related, between 14 and 45 per-

cent had been assigned the LLPDD diagnosis. These
figures came from studies conducted by members of the
LLPDD committee. When we multiplied their percentages by the total number of premenopausal women there
are likely to be in the United States, we came up with a
very conservative estimate of five hundred thousand. We
were not just worried about what *might* happen; we were
worried about what had already happened. This time,
Gold did not refute the point.

Gold also blatantly contradicted herself on the "Donahue" and "Midday" shows just weeks apart. On "Donahue," she had fully agreed that research had revealed no
hormonal link to what was being called LLPDD and that
hormone treatments did not help women who were labeled in this way. For reasons about which I can only
speculate, on "Midday" Gold completely reversed her position on a hormonal link.

On "Midday," Gold also said, "Men have circadian
rhythms that are daily," but she did not explain why men's
cycles do not appear as a mental disorder in the *DSM*.
Why should daily mood changes not be mental disorders
if monthly ones are? Is this clear evidence of gender bias
in the manual? Many studies provide evidence that men
have mood cycles, and Gloria Steinem has suggested this
perspective: "Since in women's 'difficult' days before the
onset of the menstrual period, the female hormone is at
its lowest ebb, women are in those few days the most like
what men are like *all month long*." Certainly, men's average
level of aggression is far higher than that of women. Even
Gold and her colleagues pointed out in their review of the
research that anger, which is an LLPDD criterion, tends
to be regarded as normal in men but pathological in
women and that men experience changes in mood that are

as intense as those in women. They explicitly questioned "the rationale for establishing as a psychiatric disease entity one hormonally related set of symptoms characteristic only of women." (As someone asked me, "If women's hormonally based changes that upset women are called a mental illness, isn't men's baldness—which is caused by changes in testosterone level and is upsetting to many men— a mental illness?") Perhaps such considerations led to the committee's inability to agree on a recommendation for the *DSM*. Years ago, it occurred to me that, rather than warn that women mustn't be allowed to fly airplanes, because being premenstrual might impair their piloting abilities, it might make more sense to prevent men from flying planes altogether, because one knows when women are premenstrual, but men might crash the aircraft any time. This somewhat tongue-in-cheek observation is not valid in light of the evidence that men have cyclical changes of mood and behavior, but it seems valid from the standpoint of men's greater aggressiveness (see Chapter 6 on DDPD). In fact, a recent *New York Times* writer reported a federal investigation showing that male pilots' tempers often lead to airplane crashes.

There were distortions, lies, and unexplained reversals of positions. On "Donahue," Gold claimed that they were "not moving [LLPDD] into the manual. All we have done is . . . moved [it] to Depression Unspecified." She did not tell the audience that "Depression Unspecified" *is* in the manual's main text, where only fully proven diagnoses are supposed to go. In an interview, a "DSM-IV administrator" evidently claimed that it would not go into the main text. Furthermore, as anti-LLPDD activist Dianne Corlett wrote to ask the *DSM* authors, was depression moved from fourth place up to first place in the LLPDD criteria list to justify listing the category in the main text as a depressive disorder? I began to call the whole sequence of events PMSgate. Here are a few more PMSgate incidents.

Top *DSM* and APA personnel knew very well that LLPDD was difficult, if not impossible, to recognize (how could it be otherwise when there is no evidence that it even exists?), and such difficulty naturally paves the way for its misuse and abuse, but that did not stop them from advocating its inclusion. Charlotte Grimes reported, for instance, that APA spokeswoman Diane Pennessi could not "find a way to explain it [the category]," but she didn't say how she expected therapists could understand and use it.

Many *DSM* Task Force members claimed that antidepressants help women with LLPDD, whatever it is, but they did not produce evidence either that these drugs worked any better than placebos or that the women in the studies to which they were referring were depressed only just before their periods.

Work group member and PMS researcher Jean Endicott told a reporter that women with PMDD-depression differ from women with other kinds of depression (hence implying that they should be categorized and treated differently) because "women with PMDD do not respond to all antidepressants." But exactly that is true of women and men with variously caused depressions. Most people know someone who sought help for depression and had to try one antidepressant drug after another before finding one that seemed to work for them, if indeed they found one that worked at all. It teaches us nothing about "PMDD" for antidepressants to be helpful to women who are depressed at times other than premenstrually. As noted by psychologist Jane Ussher, a researcher from University College London who has been studying PMS since the 1980s, "Women are being given drugs with often serious

side effects that are no more effective than placebos ...
[increasingly, antidepressants]. It seems to be a continuation of the 1960s and 1970s, when women who expressed
unhappiness were given antidepressants.... There was a
backlash against this, but it now seems to be returning
through the back door with PMS."

Two more PMSgate remarks are worth noting. One is
Allen Frances's admission to me that "Some members of
the [LLPDD] committee felt it should all go in the main
text, and those who read [the research] with a, shall we
say, critical eye felt it shouldn't." Clearly, Frances understood that those who had thought carefully about the research had concluded that it was not a valid category, and
yet he went on publicly and intensively to lead the push
to include it in the main text. The other comment came
from the APA's research director, Harold Pincus, who
claimed that the category of LLPDD will actually "help
women who *think* they have PMS find that they *don't* have
it but are depressed," a statement that is totally unjustified
by any systematic study.

The PMSgate stories even include one about a "mole."
At the busiest time of my work opposing LLPDD, I received a phone call from a young man who identified himself by name and said he was an undergraduate majoring
in history. He told me he planned to write his senior thesis
the following year about *DSM* and wanted to know if he
could look at the correspondence between the *DSM* people and me. In one of my published articles, I had offered
to make that correspondence available to anyone who asked,
and I told this student that I would be pleased to do so and
was glad that a history major was interested in this subject.
In the fall of 1993, he told me he would be making a trip
to a city near my home and asked if he could come and
see the documents. I agreed and offered to pick him up

from the train station if he wished and said I would like to help him as much as I could. He suddenly sounded rather standoffish and said he would not need to be picked up. When he arrived at my home, he wanted to see the correspondence immediately and asked to take it out to photocopy. I agreed, asking that he keep it in chronological order (he did not). When he returned, I asked if he had any questions. It struck me that he seemed rather cold and formal, in view of the fact that I had allowed him to come to my home and inspect any of my *DSM* papers. I asked exactly what his thesis would be about, and he looked uncomfortable (which I attributed to his not yet knowing what tack he would take—I have seen many students unduly embarrassed by not knowing what their position would be) and said he didn't know yet but would probably focus on the medicalization of mental illness. He said the only question he wanted to ask me was why I thought the *DSM* people were acting as they were. I told him what I was telling everyone: that I thought some genuinely believed they were helping people, that some wanted power and money, and that some did not know how to understand scientific research. As he left, I wished him luck with his work, told him to feel free to contact me if he needed any further information, and asked him to send me what he wrote. I thought no more about him until the beginning of 1994, when it once crossed my mind that I had heard nothing from him. Soon afterward, a newspaper reporter who was doing a story about *DSM-IV* told me that Allen Frances had urged her to speak to his nephew, who was writing his thesis about the manual. I immediately thought of this student, told her his name, and confirmed with her—and later, with the student's thesis supervisor and the student himself—that he was indeed Frances's nephew.

I would have done nothing differently had I known about the connection, but it did feel strange not to have been informed. I was told that historians do not have ethical standards that involve disclosing their conflicts of interest or their biases to people whom they ask to give them information. As I pointed out to the thesis supervisor, however, although such behavior may not technically be unethical, it is sleazy and runs the risk of making all of us researchers look bad. At the urging of his supervisor, the student sent me a copy of his thesis in the summer of 1994. It is an error-filled piece of work masquerading as intellectual history but amounting to an apologia for his uncle and his uncle's cronies. I describe some of his errors in my Notes (pp. 306-308), but here I shall just mention three that he could have avoided by asking me. One was that he claimed mistakenly that most of the people protesting the misogynist categories were Canadian. In fact, most were from the United States. In another, he asserted that "a group organized by Caplan" had planned a particular meeting about PMS. Not only had I not organized that group but I had not even heard of it until it had planned its discussion meeting and then contacted me to ask me to be a speaker. Of such unchecked errors is false history made all the time, I suppose. The student also used the same kind of insinuating language his uncle and colleagues used to refer to people on our side of the debate. For instance, he said that I had "engineered" *Ms* magazine to feature LLPDD, when, had he asked, I could have told him that I had only contacted *Ms* staff with the same information and in the same way as I had dozens of other reporters, many of whom ably resisted being "engineered" by me. His choice of that term suggested both something unsavory about me and something spineless about *Ms* magazine staff. I would have been concerned about what his thesis suggested about the quality of research, the politics, and the morality of college students, had I not taught so many fine ones myself and had I not known how much he mirrored his uncle's group.

One last example of PMSgate I find especially perplexing. Psychiatrist Nada Stotland, who had often taken courageous stands on women's issues within the APA, was a member of Judith Gold's LLPDD committee. I had been told that she believed that PMDD should have no place in *DSM-IV*. When I spoke with her on the telephone in May of 1993, she confirmed that this was her position. However, her position varied from one moment to the next, if the media reports can be believed. I know that the media can seriously distort what anyone says, so in the following description I do not know whether to assume that Stotland took very different positions at different times or that some or all of the reporters misquoted her. What I do know is that I was unable to find any sign—whether in letters to the editor or in corrections printed in newspapers—that she wanted to take a consistent position and clarify it publicly.

Betsy Lehman quoted Stotland in the *Boston Globe* as expressing concern that "the listing may harm women and stunt research into the effects of the menstrual cycle," and British reporter Gail Vines wrote that Stotland feared no distinction would be made between "a vast array of premenstrual symptoms that affect most women to some degree and the severe 'psychiatric' symptoms." However, yet another reporter—Marilyn Chase of the *Wall Street Journal*—portrayed her as defending the inclusion of PMDD in the handbook by calling opponents of the category "alarmists" and suggesting that the category would reduce misdiagnosis and encourage relevant research. The way Chase presented Stotland's position is consistent with Paula

Span's quoting of Stotland in a *Washington Post* story: " 'People *knew* 200 years ago that you treat people with leeches,' Stotland philosophizes, 'and 100 years from now people will be chuckling about what we do. . . . It's only religion that's black-and-white; science is compromise.' " Now, that direct quotation warrants some careful consideration. First of all, it is disconcerting that Stotland would treat the potential misdiagnosis of at least half a million women in such a cavalier way. Furthermore, science is not supposed to involve the kinds of compromises on political and financial grounds that this controversy has involved. In honest, carefully done scientific work, there is *no* compromise on stringent requirements for the conduct and interpretation of research. To base a major policy decision on shoddy science has never been acceptable. Stotland's turnaround in suggesting that what is clearcut is religion, rather than science, is clever and interesting but inappropriate for a member of a body that repeatedly makes public claims about the scientific basis of its decisions.

Judith Gold had taken me off her LLPDD mailing list, but someone who was still on it sent me a copy of a memo that Gold had written, in which she spelled out various options for the category. These ranged from "including it under Conditions of Medical Significance, *but not a psychiatric disorder*" (my italics) to listing it in the *DSM-IV* under "Mood Disorder Not Otherwise Specified." The first of those alternatives would not have been objectionable. I do not know when the idea of listing it in the main text under Mood Disorder changed to listing it under Depressive Disorder, which was the final decision. And that decision seems curious, because one need not even be depressed in order to fit the PMDD description, but one is required to show a mood change of some sort. In another memo, Gold made the curious announcement to her subcommittee that the LLPDD label was to be changed yet again, this time back to "Premenstrual Dysphoric Disorder." The rationale she gave for this was that it would "reflect data showing that the etiology of the symptom pattern may not be due to the hormones of the luteal phase." This seemed strange because the very word *premenstrual* naturally implies hormonal changes. More effective in avoiding such an implication would have been a title such as "Predictably Patterned Mood Changes."

As noted, after many months of reading research reports and writing a paper summarizing them, Gold's subcommittee had been unable to reach a consensus about what to recommend. When I obtained a copy of their paper, I found that in their summary, they described the existing research as "preliminary" and filled with methodological problems. They also pointed out that the research specifically relevant to the criteria of PMDD/LLPDD was only beginning to appear. In regard to this last point, there were mountains of studies about "premenstrual syndrome," which has been defined and described in dozens of different ways (see Anne Fausto-Sterling's book *Myths of Gender* for a brilliant discussion of the problems with that research), including many sets of criteria that deal exclusively with physical symptoms such as bloating and breast tenderness and therefore have nothing to do with mental disorder. The LLPDD subcommittee had recognized that the vast majority of existing research was completely or largely unrelated to mental disorder. But as *Washington Post* reporter Paula Span wrote, this was not the first time that the APA had made a decision with enormous consequences even though it was not solidly grounded: "The trustees of the American Psychiatric Association have more than once decided that hundreds of thousands of people have a form of mental illness and then, some years later, decided that they don't after all."

How did Gold's subcommittee deal with the failure to reach a consensus among themselves? Someone—perhaps either Gold or Allen Frances—decided to choose two people who were not experts on PMS and who were not on the committee, psychiatrists Nancy Andreasen and A. John Rush, to decide the fate of LLPDD. This was particularly ironic and inappropriate, because the APA had proudly and repeatedly pointed out that it had selected PMS experts to form its LLPDD subcommittee and had made sure they were all women. I suspect that the all-female composition was intended to make it more difficult to oppose the category, because the APA could argue that the category was not dangerous for women because its whole LLPDD group was composed of women. (What was not widely publicized was that one group member was the subject of an investigation by her dean on charges of impropriety in conducting her PMS research and was reprimanded by him formally and in writing.) In fact, both Andreasen and Rush had close connections to *DSM-III-R* Task Force head Robert Spitzer, who has always been a major advocate of a premenstrual mental disorder: Andreasen had coauthored published work with Spitzer and served with him on two *DSM-III-R* committees, and Rush had served on a *DSM-III-R* committee with Spitzer and had also published work about depression. This points to significant conflicts of interest because of the work both people had done with Spitzer. Furthermore, Rush's particular interest in depression prevents him from being a disinterested decision maker but does make it unsurprising (though scientifically unwarranted) that PMDD is listed in the main text under Depressive Disorders, even though the LLPDD committee had not even suggested in their massive literature review that depression was a particularly relevant classification for it. Not only is it scientifically unwarranted, because researchers have not been able to implicate the premenstrual phase as a time when depression is particularly likely to occur, but it also makes no practical sense, because one need not be depressed in order to fit the PMDD criteria. Psychiatrist Sally Severino, an LLPDD committee member and PMS researcher and early advocate of LLPDD, was quoted by reporter Gail Vines in *New Scientist* as saying that the research does not justify listing the category under "Depression." In view of all of this, it is particularly disturbing that the primary—indeed, virtually the only—psychiatric treatment Gold has publicly recommended is antidepressant drugs, a recommendation that surely warms the hearts of the pharmaceutical companies that fund research on PMS and LLPDD (see Chapter 8 for more discussion of this issue). As an added twist, an LLPDD committee member has been quoted as saying that Andreasen and Rush did not even consult with that committee before making their recommendation.

When asked about the two people who made the final recommendation, those in the *DSM* hierarchy tried to avoid disclosing Andreasen's and Rush's identities. In fact, in a telephone conversation with me on March 12, 1993, Allen Frances refused to tell me who the two people were, explaining that if he told me, they would be flooded with questions. Of course, anyone who agrees to make decisions with far-reaching impact ought to be open to questions about what they have done and ought to be identified so that they can be held accountable for their actions. After several weeks spent trying to conceal their identities, however, Frances—or someone—finally revealed them to reporter Tori deAngelis of the American Psychological Association's newspaper, the *Monitor*. Perhaps deAngelis's informant yielded because of repeated questions from media people about who had been given the power to make the recommendation.

In April, a National Public Radio producer called me to say that she wanted to arrange for an NPR debate about LLPDD between Judith Gold and me. I told her I felt the public had a right to know about the issues, but I had been increasingly concerned that, by appearing on shows with Gold, I was helping to provide airtime for the serious distortions of truth and outright lies that she and other *DSM* people were spreading, because it takes much more time to explain a serious distortion or refute a lie than the producers on most shows had been willing to allow. I said that I would be willing to appear but wanted to be assured that I would have time to make full replies. I also said that I did not want to debate Judy Gold anymore, because I had learned from experience that she was willing to lie. Sometime later, the producer called me back and gave me the following report. She had phoned APA headquarters and spoken with John Blamphin, public affairs director. When she told him about the show they were planning, he suggested that they invite Judith Gold. The producer replied that I had said I would not appear with her because she had lied. With admirable candor, according to the producer, Blamphin made no attempt to cover up for Gold but did offer the explanation that when people are "under pressure, they sometimes leave out parts of the truth."

I had decided to telephone both Blamphin and Allen Frances back on March 12 to express my concerns, the same conversation in which Frances refused to disclose Andreasen's and Rush's identities. As I told him, I felt it was doing women no good for this whole process to have become so adversarial, and I wondered if by talking reasonably together, he and I might find a way to deal with the issue. At the beginnings of our conversations, I told both Blamphin and Frances that I would be taking verbatim notes of what they said so as not to misquote them, and both said that was fine. In my conversation with Blamphin, I said that many people were alarmed by the huge number of women that LLPDD would be used to pathologize. His reply—"500,000 is not that many"—caught me by surprise. I said, "I beg your pardon," and he repeated, "500,000 is not that many—when you think how many women there are in the country." I could only imagine what a public outcry there would have been had the APA tried to pathologize half a million men in one fell swoop.

In my conversation with Frances, I told him that I wanted to ask him the question that had been put to me hundreds of times by that point: "Since your LLPDD experts' subcommittee couldn't even reach an agreement, and since in their own report they concluded that the research was very preliminary and filled with methodological problems, and since labeling women as premenstrually mentally disordered has already been shown to harm many women, why is there this push to keep it in the manual?" His response was, "I really think some women benefit from the PMDD category," but this man who had claimed that his task force's decisions would be based on scientific research acknowledged readily that he had no evidence to support his opinion. When I asked, "But what about the harm that has been done to women? Is there any evidence that more women have been helped than harmed by this category?" his reply was a breathtaking denial of what scientific research can do. "There's no way of knowing that," he said.

In regard to the question of harm to women, even after

I had told various task force members the stories of harm that had been done to women by describing them as premenstrually mentally ill (examples of which are described in detail later in this chapter), Frances and Gold continued to tell the media (see Chapter 9) that Gold's group had found no evidence of harm. The group's lengthy report includes no sign that they attempted a computer search or a survey of psychiatrists or gynecologists to find out whether any harm had been done by its placement in *DSM-III-R* (in fact, they wrote, "The potential occupational, social and forensic risks of having such a diagnosis in the nomenclature are unknown"), although evidence of such harm is easy to find. The fastest production of such evidence came to me from a journalist who, while I waited briefly on the phone, checked the Lexus database and found a child custody case in which a husband was claiming that he should get the children because his soon-to-be ex-wife was premenstrually mentally ill. Although in that case the judge had been sagacious enough to declare that the woman's medical records could not be entered as evidence, such decisions are up to the individual judge. In another case, the judge had allowed the issue of PMS to be part of a custody hearing. Furthermore, as I told *DSM* executives, I had received reports from women all over North America whose husbands were abusing them but who dared not leave because the men had threatened to claim in court that the women were premenstrually mentally ill and therefore should not have custody of their children.

Also during our talk, Frances dismissed my work in protesting the LLPDD category as "grandstanding" and speculated, as though he were my therapist, about what "stake" I had in objecting both to LLPDD and to other dangers in the mental health system. He explicitly accused me of having distorted what he and his colleagues had said. In reply, I asked if he had heard or seen any tapes of what I had said in public statements. He admitted that he had not and then acknowledged that perhaps he shouldn't have accused me without knowing what I had really said. He also sounded angry at me for having made public what he considered "private communications," that is, his letters to me. I reminded him that when he asked me to join the *DSM* committees, I had said that I would do so but that if I was uncomfortable about the process, I would feel free to resign and to speak publicly about it, and that he had agreed to this condition.

As a result of a March 12 column Michele Landsberg wrote in the *Toronto Star* about LLPDD, I received offers of help with the protest from about a dozen women, including a biology student, a housewife, a professional health worker, a writer, and some businesswomen. We met several times, and during one meeting in the late spring, I told the group that the *DSM* Task Force's recommendation to retain LLPDD had gone forward to the APA's Legislative Assembly, which was scheduled to vote on it in May during the APA convention in San Francisco. We decided to send information directly to all of the approximately 225 members of the Assembly and the APA Board. One woman in our group, Kathryn Morgan, University of Toronto Professor of Philosophy and Women's Studies, suggested that our information be focused on the impact that approving LLPDD would have on individual psychiatrists and on the APA as a body. We knew that APA groups in the past had not been persuaded by information about poor research bases for diagnoses and about dangers of particular categories, so we thought it might be useful to point out the likely legal ramifications of the proposed move. We prepared a paper headed "Before You Vote on the DSM-IV Proposal About Premenstrual Syndrome, Please Read This," and I quote some excerpts from it here. The paper began as follows:

> If the proposal to classify a version of premenstrual syndrome in the *DSM-IV* as a mental illness is approved, psychiatrists and the American Psychiatric Association itself will be the targets of lawsuits. These will be sources of enormous financial and emotional drain, as well as public embarrassment, to some of you as individual practitioners and to the Association and the profession of psychiatry as a whole.

> It will almost inevitably lead to an increase in the cost of malpractice insurance, especially since—according to the figures of your *DSM-IV*'s premenstrual disorder committee—at least half a million North American women will be so classified. As committee chair Dr. Judith Gold has said publicly, they expect that the number of women who will receive this diagnosis will be about the same as the number of people diagnosed as depressed—a massive number.

Lawsuits are rarely filed until years after harm occurs, partly because the victims are usually so drained and debilitated from the harm that most of their energy goes into simply trying to manage their daily lives and partly because it can take time for them to realize that they have cause for a lawsuit.

We told the Legislative Assembly members that we would provide information about four issues, including legal liability implications related to each one:

1. the kinds of documented **harm** already done to women through use of this psychiatric diagnosis
2. a brief summary (mostly in the words of your own *DSM* Task Force's premenstrual disorder subcommittee's own research review) of what the **research** on PMS reveals in regard to having some form of PMS in the *DSM*
3. a brief description of the **process** by which the current proposal to include a form of PMS in the upcoming edition of the *DSM* was reached—and the deeply disturbing and now widely publicized features of that process
4. a short summary of the **pro and con arguments** related to the proposal

We began the section on harm by stating that lawsuits will be based on harm to women as a result of receiving this kind of diagnosis, and we explained that significant harm had already come to many women. We felt it was crucial to describe the harm for two reasons. First of all, harm matters, in and of itself. Decision makers need to be aware of the harm that their decisions can cause. And harm is all the more worrying if the concept that causes the harm has not even been proven to label a real phenomenon of mental illness or if it has not been shown that people can be helped by the label. For example, many people find it easier to understand the dangers of the old psychiatric category of drapetomania, which was described as a psychiatric disorder of slaves who tried to run away, than of sexist categories that are dangerous and have not been proven to exist. In our paper for the Legislative Assembly, as examples of LLPDD's harm, we began with the child custody dispute and then gave these others:

- Employers' claims that a woman's premenstrual

psychiatric disorder justified firing her from her job or not hiring her

- Documented suicide attempts or other severe side effects from antidepressant medication that was given when women reported having premenstrual mood changes (in cases reported up to now, the antidepressants not only caused severe harm but also failed to help the symptoms that were described as premenstrual)
- Physicians' failure to diagnose painful or deteriorating physical problems (such as worsening sexually transmitted diseases causing pain, scarring, and infertility) because they have focused on the woman's emotional symptoms that were secondary to the physical pain and therefore focused on "treating" their alleged premenstrual illness
- Increases in anxiety and/or depression due to being labeled as mentally ill

In regard to doctors' failure to diagnose physical problems because they are focusing on emotional symptoms, a specific story will illustrate how dangerous this can be. A woman in her early thirties sought help from a series of physicians because she had intense physical pain for some days before each menstrual period. She had not had such pain from the time of her first period; it had begun when she was a young adult. She was repeatedly told that there was nothing physically wrong with her, that the pain must be emotionally caused. At one point, she specifically asked a doctor to check her for infection, and he said that he had done so and that she had none. As the years went by and the excruciating physical pain continued, the woman became understandably more and more depressed and anxious. From time to time, she went to additional doctors, including psychiatrists, but this did not help, because they would focus on her depression and anxiety and use those symptoms to "prove" that her problems were simply emotional. Finally, she had to have surgery for an unrelated physical problem, and when the incision was made, the surgeon found masses of old scar tissue due to infection. He removed some of the scar tissue; it was impossible to take out the rest. An antibiotic speedily cleared up the years-old infection, but the woman is left with a great deal of scarring, which the doctors now acknowledge had been causing her pain all along, and it is unlikely that she will be able to bear children.

In regard to the harm of increasing patients' depression or anxiety by classifying them as mentally ill, we explained in our position paper that a therapist's labeling of a patient as mentally ill is legally actionable when research fails to justify applying that label for that individual case or when it fails to justify classifying such a problem as a mental illness at all.

We were trying to keep our position paper reasonably brief, so there were other kinds of harm that we did not mention. For instance, there is no safeguard to keep the label from being applied wholesale to large numbers of women. In the introductory material before the criteria for LLPDD are listed, psychiatrists are told that they should have women keep a checklist of their symptoms for two months before they assign this diagnosis. However, under the criteria one finds the note that women should be given this label if they experienced the symptoms in "most" menstrual cycles during the previous year and that the symptoms should be regularly present during the week before the period starts and perhaps a few days after the bleeding begins. If a woman must only keep a checklist for two months but is supposed to describe every month from the preceding year, then retrospective reports will make up the bulk of the information she gives her doctor. This is worrying, because, as the *DSM* authors acknowledge in the handbook, women tend to describe symptoms they regard as premenstrual as less severe when they are experiencing them than when they try to recall them later on. There will, therefore, be a built-in tendency for inflated numbers of women to receive this diagnosis. Furthermore, no one seems to have determined how many therapists take care to ensure that the symptoms are *only* experienced just before and at the beginning of the period.

Another source of harm due to the therapist's wide latitude for judging women relates to the therapist's judgment of the severity of the symptoms. All of the features that involve moods and feelings are supposed to be "marked": "marked depression," "marked irritability," and so on. Obviously, what is marked irritability to one therapist may appear to be only moderate or minimal irritability to another. In view of the pressure on women in our culture not to show irritation, anger, or depression, one cannot help but worry about whether any display of irritability or other "unfeminine," "negative" feelings might be too readily considered to be "marked."

An especially serious source of harm comes from the claim by Gold's group that antidepressant medication is the one psychiatric treatment they have to offer. Aside from the lack of research to support their usefulness for women who complain of severe PMS, antidepressants (and most recently, Prozac) have long been used to mask problems that women have due to harassment, violence, or various forms of sexist treatment. That does not mean that the drugs do not make some women feel better, whether their depression comes only premenstrually or at other times as well; but the fact that crack and heroin give many people some relief from the oppression and misery of our inner cities does not make us eager to prescribe those drugs for them. In the latter case, we see clearly that it is morally wrong to use drugs to cover up underlying social problems and divert their victims' attention from them.

Everyday kinds of harm include men's and women's dismissal and trivializing of women's legitimate concerns and grievances as "just PMS." Hand in hand with those practices goes the covering up of men's role in creating interpersonal conflict and abuse. At the very worst, both women and men blame women for their own abuse, claiming that their "PMS" behavior provokes it. In a general sense, the use of the LLPDD category tends to deflect attention away from situational problems, such as abusive partners or low-paying jobs, that could be leading to women's upsetting mood changes. In her 1994 master's thesis research, Heather Nash found that the presence of this category in the *DSM* significantly increases the frequency with which people of both sexes attribute disturbing behavior in women to the menstrual cycle. As Nash wrote, "gender-neutral emotions become woman-only experiences as soon as they fall under the title of a menstrual cycle disorder." And summarizing the findings from her study, she concluded, "Despite the fact that the diagnosis is only supposed to be given in the most severe cases, men and women in the general public will see their female employers, professors, friends and acquaintances, and their mothers as suffering from it when they are given knowledge of the diagnostic criteria."

In our position paper's section on research, we wrote:

> Judicial decisions like those in the Dalkon Shield and Meme breast implant cases make it absolutely clear that both individual physicians and groups that endorse particular actions (such as assignment of di-

agnostic categories) can be held liable for harm **especially when the research does not justify the action.** This is the case for placing "Premenstrual Dysphoric Disorder" (PMDD) in the *DSM-IV.* The *DSM-IV* Task Force has a committee on PMDD that met and reviewed the research for several years.

Here we quoted from that committee's conclusion about the sparseness and the poor quality of the relevant research. Then we described an extremely important study that had recently been published:

> The most relevant and methodologically sound study was conducted by Sheryle Gallant, Jean Hamilton, and their colleagues and demonstrated without question that the category of PMDD is neither valid nor helpful to women. They asked women who said they had severe premenstrual symptoms and women who said they had none to keep a checklist of the specific PMDD criteria, just as physicians are supposed to do before assigning the PMDD label to a patient. They found that the women's checklist responses failed to distinguish the two groups. The ability of the checklist to distinguish *at least* between women who have no PMS and women who report severe symptoms would have been essential to supporting the validity of this category. Indeed, if the *DSM-IV* spokespeople's claim is true, that only a small percentage of women with PMS will get the psychiatric diagnosis, then the checklist should even have been able to make the finer distinction between women reporting mild or moderate and women reporting severe symptoms. But the criteria chosen for PMDD fail even to allow clinicians to distinguish the severe cases from women who do not complain of premenstrual problems at all.

Even more astonishing is that Gallant and her colleagues had also asked some *men* to fill out the checklist, and even their answers did not differ from those of the women who had described themselves as having severe PMS. Thus, the key study to test whether there *is* such a thing as PMDD as described by the APA had actually been done, and it showed clearly that PMDD is definitely *not* a valid category. That is very dramatic proof that the APA's big push to classify PMDD as a mental illness is unjustified.

We do not fault Gold's group for failing to produce excellent research on PMS or PMDD, for that was not their task. Indeed, in our book *Thinking Critically About Research on Sex and Gender*, my son, Jeremy B. Caplan, and I listed many of the large number of reasons that it is so difficult to conduct good, conclusive research on this topic. In so doing, we followed in the footsteps of many others who have identified such obstacles (such as Anne Fausto-Sterling, Mary Brown Parlee, Michele Harrison, and Carol Tavris.) The fault of the *DSM* Task Force itself, more than Gold's group which did *not* make a recommendation, is to have ignored these significant obstacles in reaching its decision. And the fault of some of the members of Gold's group, including Gold herself, was to defend the Andreasen-Rush recommendation even though the group had not been able to agree on it. Of Gold's work group members, Severino is noteworthy for her integrity in being honest about her position and the reasons for it, even when it has meant disagreeing with her colleagues.

We next addressed the fact that the task force was recommending that PMDD appear not only in the provisional appendix but also in the main text, which is supposedly reserved for fully accepted labels, under "Depressive Disorders." We pointed out:

This increases the risk that the many *real* causes of women's depression will be ignored because it will be too easy to attribute such depression to hormones—again increasing the risk of physicians overlooking serious problems and being held accountable. The actual PMDD criteria show that one need not even be depressed at all in order to receive that diagnosis. As long as a woman is *either* depressed *or* anxious *or* irritable *or* emotionally labile *and* has four physical symptoms such as breast tenderness and bloating, *she will fit the description of this "mental illness."*

Next, we tried to draw the Assembly's attention to the likelihood that sex discrimination would be alleged in future lawsuits:

Research has shown that men have hormonally-based cycles in their moods (as PMDD committee head Dr. Judith Gold has publicly acknowledged), but the *DSM* Task Force does not plan to classify this as a mental illness—making it dead easy to prove sex discrimination.

The next issue we addressed was that of treatment:

The only psychiatric treatment the *DSM* Task Force members have suggested for PMDD is the use of antidepressants. Again, since research in that area is primarily poorly designed and therefore invalid, and since reviews of that research have shown that antidepressants work no better than placebos for symptoms described as premenstrual, the issue of doctors' accountability again arises. This issue is compounded by the serious side effects many women have suffered from psychotropic drugs *at the same time as those drugs have failed to alleviate the symptoms the women report as premenstrual.* Furthermore, researchers' attempts to find higher rates of depression premenstrually than at other times of the cycle have never succeeded; in fact, the research shows that, contrary to folk wisdom, depression is least likely to occur premenstrually.

An additional ethical and legal issue related to the research is that, as Dr. Gold has publicly acknowledged, hormonal treatments for premenstrual mood problems do not work. Therefore, the application of a diagnostic label that clearly implicates the hormones (i.e., "Premenstrual" disorder rather than, say, "Depression" or "Anxiety disorder") is unjustified by the research. Harm to a woman because of the PMDD label can be related partly to the absence of a research base for the hormonal connection. And this absence of research is a far more powerful argument in court than the testimony of individual doctors claiming that "We just *know* there must be a hormonal link."

Our last two comments about the research were focused on the strange plan to put the title, PMDD, in the main text but its criteria in the provisional appendix for categories needing further study, and also on a final risk related to lawsuits:

Many people have wondered why they would put the label in the main text but the criteria in the appendix. As one person said, "It looks like the *DSM* Task Force is so certain that there *is* such a phenomenon that they put the label in the fully-approved section, but after all these years of research they still don't know what it consists of, so they have to have the criteria stay in a provisional

appendix." When Task Force head Dr. Allen
Frances was asked on March 12, 1993, about the
reason for this split, he said: "That's what the
precedent was in the *DSM-III-R*." All decisions
about the *DSM-IV* are supposed to be made on the
basis of good research, not on the weak grounds
of "precedent."

Other evidence that could become relevant in legal
proceedings is that members of the Task Force and
the PMDD committee have said publicly that they
know the research does not justify the proposed
action.

As Table 1 shows, even a therapist who might intentionally choose to use the LLPDD (now PMDD) diagnosis
from the appendix rather than from the main text *because
the appendix is only for provisional categories* will find *in
the appendix* that a formal five-digit code (300.90) is provided for coding purposes, making it seem well validated
and official.

In the section about the decision-making process, we
summarized many of the disturbing aspects of the process
that were described earlier in this chapter. We also reported an encouraging and quite dramatic development:

> In an unprecedented step, a major hospital (Wom-
> en's College Hospital in Toronto) has issued a press
> release stating its opposition to this category, and its
> psychiatrist-in-chief, APA Ontario branch executive
> member Dr. Howard Book, has been interviewed
> by the media about his support for that opposition.

To my knowledge, this is the only known instance of a
hospital taking a stand against a particular category of psychiatric diagnosis.

In our last section, on the pros and cons of the issue, we dealt with each of the *DSM* Task Force's and LLPDD subcommittee's claims:

1. They claim that they are not calling all women with PMS mentally ill but only a very small percentage of them.
HOWEVER, if we put together their claim that only 3% of women with PMS ever seek help, plus their own research showing that between 14% and *45%* of women seeking help for PMS will be given the *psychiatric label of PMDD*, we come up with a very conservative estimate of 500,000 women in the U.S. alone who would be so classified. Although they have repeatedly denied this in public, those figures are reported in their own publication, the *DSM-IV Update* of January/February 1993, and the 45% figure was also found in a study by Jensvold.

We then reported Blamphin's comment that five hundred thousand women was not very many. Continuing with our response to their first claim, we wrote:

FURTHERMORE, they point out that the criteria specify that the woman must have not just depression but "marked" depression, so they believe there is no danger that the category will be overused. However, as you know, use of the label is entirely up to the clinician's interpretation and discretion. There is no central registry that ensures that only a tiny percentage of women will receive the label. No doctor is prevented from assigning it to more than a certain fraction of their patients.

A quick look at Table 1 reveals further opportunities for application of the label to large numbers of women. In Section D, therapists are told that they should not diagnose a woman as PMDD if her disturbance is "merely the exacerbation of . . . another disorder" *although* it *may be superimposed* on another disorder. Any honest clinician will confess that, especially in the early stages of evaluation of a patient, it is difficult if not impossible to tell whether one disturbance is merely an exacerbation of another or whether it is "superimposed" on it. In Section E, the therapist is told that the criteria "are confirmed by" prospective daily self-ratings for at least two monthly cycles but then is given permission to go ahead and make the diagnosis "provisionally" *without* obtaining this confirmation.

We then addressed the *DSM* authors' second major claim:

> **2. They say that their reason for doing this is "to help women."**
> *HOWEVER*, on March 12, Dr. Frances was asked for evidence that classifying PMS as a mental illness has helped women and replied, "I really think some women benefit from the PMDD category" but said that he had no evidence of this. When asked, "Is there any evidence that more women have been helped than harmed by this category?" he replied, "There's no way of knowing that."

In closing, we wrote:

> To put this whole issue in an appropriate context, *IF* the APA had reported that research showed that both Blacks and Whites have hormonally-based mood cycles but that they planned only to pathologize those of Blacks, we would cry "Racism!" And we

would be right. This move is as sexist as that one would be racist. It has been well-documented that the average level of men's anger and irritability— not to mention violence—is far higher than that of even most women who report having severe PMS, yet the DSM Task Force refused to consider a proposal for labeling extreme forms of rigid, traditionally "masculine" behavior as a significant problem. This, combined with the research revealing men's hormonally-based mood changes, is more fodder for lawsuits and formal complaints.

Those opposed to including PMDD in the manual are not saying that they do not believe it when women say that they have a difficult time premenstrually. What they are saying is that some women have *physical* symptoms premenstrually, and that definitely is *not* a mental illness. Then, there are women who report having mood changes premenstrually that they find upsetting. But as noted, researchers have not been able to find that mood changes are more commonly found during that part of the menstrual cycle. Furthermore, research has shown that those women who report premenstrual mood problems are more likely than other women to be in upsetting life circumstances. And the treatments that have been shown to be most helpful are changes in exercise, diet and nutrition, and self-help groups—hardly the stuff of psychiatric illness. Dr. Dodie Pirie, who runs such groups, has found through her research that one of the most important features of the groups is their reframing of the anger and irritability that the women believe is "too great"; thus, they come to understand that, as women, they have felt so ashamed of and frightened by their "negative" feelings and behavior that they have needed to attribute it to uncontrollable hormonal changes.

If women are depressed and feel they are helped by antidepressants, it is not necessary to diagnose them as having hormonally-based or "premenstrual" depression in order to help them. Categories for depression are already in the *DSM*.

We signed the paper "From: The Coalition for a Scientific and Responsible *DSM-IV*."

Shortly before the Legislative Assembly was scheduled to vote, I contacted psychiatrist Nada Stotland, who had been described to me as an influential member of the LLPDD committee. I had also been told that she had said the category did not belong in the handbook at all. In our conversation, she confirmed this but said she did not know how to stop the Assembly from voting to keep it in. I told her that I felt it would be important for someone within APA to ask the Assembly to review the concerns about LLPDD before voting on it. Stotland replied that she feared that bringing up LLPDD for discussion would create an opening for all sorts of bad things to happen, such as reinstating SDPD. Once *any DSM* issue was considered up for discussion, every proposed change might be, she said.

I was unable to be in San Francisco for the convention but was in touch with a number of opponents of LLPDD. Representatives from the San Francisco chapter of the National Organization for Women, organized by Karen Brooks, and approximately one hundred psychiatric survivors led by David Oaks, publisher of *Dendron News*, a newspaper critical of the mental health establishment, held public demonstrations against the category. They were invited to send representatives to a meeting with some of the *DSM* personnel and did so. According to Brooks, a male representative of APA told her, "We'll be sending women so you won't have to talk to men about this." A feminist psychologist I knew reported that on the way to that meeting she approached a woman psychiatrist whom I had described as agreeing with our views. She told this woman that I had suggested they make contact. She reported to me that the psychiatrist told her, "We asked Paula Caplan to join our committee, but she declined, and we don't know why." That, of course, was simply untrue; I had been on the committee but had resigned, and that was certainly by then a matter of public knowledge. This technique of trying to discredit those who disagree with them by falsely portraying them as bafflingly uncooperative has been used many times by *DSM* authors.

Psychologist Sara Edmonds, who attended the meeting, described it this way:

> The five female psychiatrists who were there, plus the head of the Legislative Assembly, . . . were basically pacifying, noncommittal, and dismissing. They said they'd already considered the issues we brought up, they didn't want the women to be labeled either, they only wanted to speak to NOW people (NOW said we are in this together [with Network Against Psychiatric Assault and Support Coalition International]) and if we knew of specific cases of women being mislabeled with this diagnosis to bring them to their attention. . . . I asked why they had moved the diagnosis into the Depressive Disorder category and they said they had done that based on their review of the literature.

The misrepresentation and the patronizing attitude of so many *DSM* participants characterized that meeting, then, as much as they have the rest of the *DSM* process.

Well after the APA convention, someone sent me a copy of the letter Gail Robinson, head of the APA's own Committee on Women, had sent to Allen Frances on April

28. In that letter, she articulately expressed nearly every reason for opposing LLPDD that we had also voiced, but apparently, the *DSM* higher-ups ignored her concerns as well.

I had assumed that the Legislative Assembly would be asked to vote on each proposed *DSM* change in turn, since each would have profound impact on so many future patients. It turned out, however, that the Assembly members were just asked to vote "yes" or "no" on the entire, massive batch of proposed changes to the manual. The extensive concerns about LLPDD and other categories were not even dignified by a few minutes of separate attention to them. The Assembly approved the proposed changes.

It then remained only for the APA Board to rubberstamp the Assembly's decision in the Board meeting in Washington, D.C., the following July, as indeed they did. A couple of days after that vote, I appeared on the "Today" show with Spitzer. When the interviewer, Katie Couric, announced that the APA had voted to consider a form of PMS a mental illness, Spitzer said that that was not what had happened. All that had occurred, he claimed, was that the APA had voted to continue to list the category in its "list of disorders that need further study," that is, the provisional appendix. He went on to say explicitly that the APA "did not move up the disorder to an official category." And when Couric asked him, "So right now is it or is it not listed as a mental disorder?" he again repeated, "It's in this limbo . . . and not listed within the full list of official categories." What flashed through my mind at first was that that was exactly the claim he had made at this stage in regard to LLPDD and the *DSM-III-R*, and I wondered whether he was again distorting the truth. My next thought, however, was that I would have about forty-five seconds of airtime, and that wouldn't be enough to explain to the viewers why they should care whether or not the category was also listed in the main text. I made a mental note to check later on the veracity of Spitzer's claim on the national television show. And indeed, Spitzer's history had repeated itself, for once again the category appears not only in the provisional appendix but also in the main text, this time under the heading of "Depressive Disorders Not Otherwise Specified." In fact, it is the first category listed under that heading. It was one more incident in the PMSgate history.

At some point in the last few months before the Board's vote, someone decided to switch the label from LLPDD back to the original 1985 label, "Premenstrual Dysphoric Disorder." As usual, there was no public explanation for the change, but I have to wonder if it was an intentional or unintentional acknowledgment of their inability to find research to back up the scientific-sounding specificity of "Late Luteal Phase." They made a few other significant changes for the *DSM-IV* listing. As noted, they moved the depression criterion up to first place. They added a new criterion, "a subjective sense of being overwhelmed or out of control," and added to the "affective lability" criterion the example of "increased sensitivity to rejection," both of which are consistent with the stereotypic view of women as overly emotional. They also noted that mea-surement of reproductive hormones circulating in the blood may be necessary, but they do this in spite of Judith Gold's committee's conclusion that there is little or no evidence that what is called PMDD is caused by changes in reproductive hormones.

What's Really Happening to These Women?

Few people complain that they are self-defeating or masochistic, unless they have been misled by experts or by friends claiming that some people actually enjoy suffering. But what about the women who say they have severe mood problems premenstrually? For some women, hormonal changes may be one factor or even the major factor in the mood changes they experience before their periods. I cannot say, however, that I believe their moods are straightforwardly and completely caused by hormonal changes, because too many major flaws have been found in researchers' attempts to demonstrate that cause-effect relationship and too many nonbiological factors have been shown to increase women's perceptions of themselves as having premenstrual emotional problems. But under no circumstances would I want to give the impression that women who say they have PMS should be ignored or disbelieved. As psychologist Mary Brown Parlee has said, to conclude that suffering is not biologically based should not be to conclude that it is not real. When people tell me they are suffering, I believe them. Once having accepted what they say, it seems to me that the greatest service one can provide is to get to the bottom of *why* they are suffering. After reading the research and interviewing women about this issue, I have come to believe that many individual or combinations of factors can culminate in women's reports that they have PMS.

When some women say they have severe PMS, they are referring only to physical symptoms, which can indeed be quite severe. These include breast tenderness and bloating. Sometimes, women mistakenly describe as "PMS" the uterine cramps that occur *during* rather than before bleeding. Uncomfortable though these may be, they do not constitute a mental illness, and they are menstrual, not *pre*menstrual problems. When women have tended to report having trouble before bleeding begins, they have named both physical and mood problems, but they have usually reported only physical ones *during* the days of bleeding. Then, as we have said, some women report in retrospect that they are only or mostly upset just before their periods, but when they keep records *at the time*, that turns out not to be the case. Similarly, when women keep records at the time, they do not describe their symptoms as being as severe as when they are asked to describe them after the fact. What is going on here? It is not that women lie but rather that, having been raised to feel they are always supposed to be cheerful and positive, they need to find excuses or explanations for their depressed, anxious, irritable, or angry moods or behavior when they can no longer conceal them. It's a way of saying, "Please don't get mad at me. I can't help it. It's just my hormones." This hypothesis is borne out by the dramatic reduction of symptoms experienced by women once they have spent some time in self-help groups where they are helped to understand the sources of their "negative" feelings and to find ways they can be comfortable dealing with them.

Other women feel depressed, angry, or irritable all month but notice it more, or feel able to excuse or justify it more, when they are premenstrual. This would not be a premenstrual mental illness either, but it does warrant some discussion. First of all, research has shown that women who say they have mood problems premenstrually are more likely than other women to be in upsetting life situations, such as abusive relationships or high-pressured work environments. Dr. Ian Tummon, an obstetrician-gynecologist and specialist in reproductive technology practicing in London, Ontario, has written an article suggesting that the term "PMS" no longer be used. He told me that when his women patients come to see him and begin their appointment by saying, "Doctor, I have terrible PMS," they never mention PMS during the rest of the session. Instead, he says, they spend the whole time talking about the way their husbands abuse them or their fourteen-year-old children won't come home at night. Many women have serious problems and deserve to be treated with respect and offered help that is to the point. Diagnosing them as mentally ill will not do the job. Giving women like these antidepressants or tranquilizers may artificially elevate their moods or suppress their anxieties but doesn't get rid of the sources of their troubles. For instance, there is a positive correlation between marital dissatisfaction and the reported intensity of premenstrual symptoms. Women must be allowed to choose drugs, of course, if they have been completely informed about the ways they work and any undesirable effects they can have, *and* if they are offered help in dealing productively with the real *causes* of their emotional upset. But labeling and drugging women should not be the treatments of choice.

Furthermore, giving a woman a psychiatric label makes it less likely that she will make changes in her nutrition, diet, and exercise or join a self-help group, and these have been shown to help enormously in cases when women describe themselves as having severe PMS. Columnist Michele Landsberg reported:

> "Just talking about their PMS with other women reduces the severity of symptoms by 40 to 50 per cent," says Dodie Pirie, a psychologist who also believes that chemical treatment is ineffective. The worst stress, she feels, is created by the lack of permission that women feel in their families to be angry, to say no, to assert themselves. "The range of acceptable feelings for women is very narrow, from bland to nurturing." Once women compare notes and see that anger and mood swings are normal, the symptoms abate.

It is not necessary for us to assume, as some have done, that women are lying about or exaggerating their mood changes in order to explain why researchers have not found more extreme mood changes premenstrually than at other times of the month, for as described above, there are understandable reasons that women tend to say that their mood problems come just before their periods. If women are depressed and want a diagnosis so that their insurance will cover their psychotherapy sessions, for instance, it is not necessary to diagnose them as having hormonally based or "premenstrual" depression in order to help them, for "Depression" is already listed in the *DSM*. As psychologist Carol Tavris has said: "If women are depressed, they should be treated for depression.... And if they have severe symptoms associated with the menstrual cycle, they should be seeing a gynecologist, not a psychiatrist" (although some gynecologists are quick to prescribe antidepressants, when self-help groups, diet, and exercise changes might help more).

One further comment about what women call PMS is in order. I believe, based on my own experience, that hormonal changes can affect one's mood and emotions. When my daughter seemed to lose interest in breastfeeding and demanded more solid food, I spent several days feeling depressed. When I noticed that I felt depressed, I then felt ashamed, because I thought that it signified my inability to let her grow up. I worried that I would ruin her emotionally because of these inappropriate feelings. Fortunately, I had to phone Diane Sacks, our pediatrician, about something else, and at the end of our conversation, she asked how I was feeling. I mentioned that I had weaned Emily and was feeling depressed. "Oh, yes," she said nonchalantly, "that's hormonal. That'll go away in a few days." I felt relieved. My feelings had been normalized, and I relaxed, knowing that I need not be alarmed. Similarly, I believe that women's hormonal changes—at various times of their cycle and like men's hormonal changes—can affect their moods. (An important and serious source of trouble for women, which has been recognized in Britain more than in North America, has been the appearance or increase of premenstrual problems in women after they have tubal ligation surgery.) However, I think the analogy of a sprained ankle is useful in understanding what happens. A person who sprains an ankle one morning may not be particularly bothered by the pain during the day, while busy at work. However, upon returning home and having to make dinner while feeling very tired, that person will probably be more sensitive and reactive to the ankle pain. And as Tavris has pointed out, chronic lower back pain can cause depression and irritability. But no one would think to call a sprained ankle or lower back pain a mental disorder. One could appropriately call them factors that can exacerbate existing depression, fear, irritability, anger, or anxiety. Thus, it seems likely that some women, for various reasons, have more trouble premenstrually than others. For some, it is possible that hormonal changes have severe effects on them, but the research shows that the situational factors that can shape women's perceptions of their premenstrual state are so powerful that it becomes difficult to know what the hormonal contribution might be. Furthermore, the failure of researchers to demonstrate hormonal causes or to demonstrate that hormonal treatments help with "PMS" suggests that it would be profitable to emphasize the way we help women learn to deal with the ways they report feeling premenstrually. Anyone experiencing uncomfortable or upsetting physical or emotional states *for whatever reason* will be helped by offers of support or help, and saying, "Your hormones are making you mentally ill" is not helpful. In spite of what the *DSM* people say, one need not declare a person mentally ill in

order to let her know that you believe her and want to
assist her in any way that she would find helpful.

A rather different aspect of women's premenstrual experience about which I am often asked is, "As a feminist,
don't you want PMDD to be an official category, so
women can kill their husbands and not have to go to jail?"
Such questioners have a twisted view of feminism, but the
use of PMS or PMDD as a defense in criminal cases does
deserve some discussion. I cannot say that I want anyone
labeled mentally ill in order to keep them out of jail, and
in any case, as Elizabeth Holtzman said when she was a
Brooklyn district attorney, "There is . . . no scientific evidence that shows women lose the ability to know right
from wrong" when they are premenstrual. Most important, PMS defenses have made great headlines but have
diverted attention from the real reasons some women have
felt desperate or frightened enough to attack or kill. The
more stories I read about women who have committed
crimes and used the PMS defense, the more I have begun
to notice a pattern (and at least one other observer of
these cases, Kathleen Kendall, shares my view). I suspect
that defense lawyers have used the PMS strategy because
they sense judges' and juries' willingness to believe that
women's hormones make them irrational or crazy, but in
the media stories I have seen in the past year about such
cases, the woman has killed or attacked a man who had
abused her for a long period of time. Lawyers may feel
that a PMS defense is more likely to be accepted than an
argument of self-defense due to a history of battering.
Until recently, courts have resisted self-defense arguments
unless the woman committed the crime in *immediate* response to battering. So if the woman had good reason to
believe that she or her children would be abused in the
future, the courts would not consider that a legitimate

defense. Irresponsible professionals appearing as expert witnesses have tried to support PMS defenses, and this helps no one. For example, in the case of a woman who stabbed a man who had beaten her in the past, Dr. Jeffrey Nisker, a gynecologist and "expert" on PMS, said he diagnosed her as having PMS but admitted he knew of no research connecting that kind of behavior with the condition. Another example of the way the defense masks women's real problems came in a newspaper article about a twenty-four-year-old woman who was said to have diminished mental capacity due to PMS. The woman was accused of having beaten her four-year-old daughter when the daughter refused to be quiet. Well into the article, however, the woman was described as a single mother of six children, and she was clearly poor because she was represented by a Legal Aid lawyer, but no one suggested *those* enormous responsibilities as sources of the kind of desperation and panic that can lead to abuse, and evidently the unnamed reporter didn't ask. In summary, then, I fear that PMS defenses probably do women more harm than good because they keep us as a society from looking at the real causes of women's problems.

The most relevant commentary I have seen on the issue was the caption of a cartoon that was mailed to me (the name of whose creator and the source of which I unfortunately cannot tell from the clipping). Under the drawing of some women and men at a cocktail party are the words of one of the women: "Mr. Dumbkauf, you think a woman shouldn't be President because her menstrual cycle would make her act crazy and want to declare war on somebody? Gee, I'm in my cycle now—as are millions of other women. Can you explain why we're not all out in the street stabbing, shooting and setting fire to people?"

6

Delusional Dominating Personality Disorder: "If This Sounds Discouraging, I'm Afraid It Is Meant To"

Since becoming aware of the pervasiveness of bias and political agendas in the shaping of the *DSM*, I had often said in public lectures that women were pathologized more than men in the handbook.* Usually, I said something like, "They call women mentally ill when they follow traditionally 'feminine' socialization (SDPD), and they say that 'female hormones' make women psychiatrically disordered. But they don't consider the results of rigid 'masculine' socialization to be a problem; they don't have a category of 'Macho Personality Disorder' or 'John Wayne Syndrome.' And they don't have a category of 'Testosterone-Based Aggression,' even though there is evidence that men are far more violent than women and that one part of this *may* be due to their hormones." After one such lecture in 1989, feminist sociologist Margrit Eichler suggested to me that we design something like "Macho Personality Disorder." Soon after, we did

*Parts of this chapter were taken from my article "How *do* they decide who is normal? The bizarre, but true tale of the *DSM* process." *Canadian Psychology/Psychologie Canadienne* 32 (1991):162–70.

just that. We called it Delusional Dominating Personality Disorder (DDPD) (Table 1 is a description of DDPD). When Margrit asked about submitting it for the *DSM-IV*, I told her that, on the basis of my exposure to the deeply entrenched sexism in the APA, I seriously doubted that they would accept it. We felt we had nothing to lose by submitting the proposal, however, and we hoped at least to draw the attention of some people to the fact that this is a very real problem. We also began to speak publicly about DDPD and found it to be an excellent consciousness-raising and thought-provoking tool.

Table 1. Delusional Dominating Personality Disorder (Proposal)

Individuals having this disorder are characterized by at least 6(?) of the following 14 criteria (note that such individuals nearly always suffer from at least one of the delusions listed):

1. Inability to establish and maintain meaningful interpersonal relationships
2. Inability to identify and express a range of feelings in oneself (typically accompanied by an inability to identify accurately the feelings of other people)
3. Inability to respond appropriately and empathically to the feelings and needs of close associates and intimates (often leading to the misinterpretation of signals from others)
4. Tendency to use power, silence, withdrawal, and/or avoidance rather than negotiation in the face of interpersonal conflict or difficulty
5. Adoption of gender-specific locus of control (belief that women are responsible for the bad things that happen to oneself, and the good things are due to one's own abilities, achievements, or efforts)
6. Excessive need to inflate the importance and achievements of oneself, males in general, or both. This is often associated with a need to deflate the importance of one's intimate female partner, females in general, or both

7. The presence of any one of the following delusions: (a) the delusion of personal entitlement to the services of (i) any woman with whom one is personally associated, (ii) females in general or males in general, (iii) both of the above; (b) the delusion that women like to suffer and be ordered around; (c) the delusion that physical force is the best method of solving interpersonal problems; (d) the delusion that sexual and aggressive impulses are uncontrollable in (i) oneself, (ii) males in general, or (iii) both of the above; (e) the delusion that pornography and erotica are identical; (f) the delusion that women control most of the world's wealth and/or power but do little of the world's work; (g) the delusion that existing inequalities in the distribution of power and wealth are a product of the survival of the fittest and, therefore, allocation of greater social and economic rewards to the already privileged are merited. (Note: The simultaneous presence of several of these delusions in one individual is common and frequently constitutes a profoundly distorted belief system.)

8. A pronounced tendency to categorize spheres of functioning and sets of behavior rigidly according to sex, e.g., belief that housework is women's work

9. A pronounced tendency to use a gender-based double standard in interpreting or evaluating situations or behavior (e.g., a man who makes breakfast sometimes is considered to be extraordinarily good, but a woman who sometimes neglects to make breakfast is considered deficient)

10. A need to affirm one's social importance by displaying oneself in the company of females who meet any three of the following criteria: (a) are conventionally physically attractive; (b) are younger than oneself; (c) are shorter in stature than oneself; (d) weigh less than oneself; (e) appear to be lower on socioeconomic criteria than oneself; (f) are more submissive than oneself

11. A distorted approach to sexuality displaying itself in one or both of these ways: (a) an excessive need for flattery about one's sexual performance and/or the size of one's genitalia; (b) an infantile tendency to equate large breasts on women with their sexual attractiveness

12. A tendency to feel inordinately threatened by women who fail to disguise their intelligence

13. An inability to derive pleasure from doing things for others

14. Emotionally uncontrolled resistance to reform efforts that are oriented toward gender equity; note that the tendency to consider oneself a "New Man" neither proves nor disproves that the patient fits within this diagnostic category and patients who fit this description should *not* be diagnosed as having obsessive-compulsive disorders, since obsessive-compulsive disorder affects only a limited part of the personality and functioning, whereas this disorder is pervasive and profound, a maladaptive organization of the entire personality.

When submitting DDPD to Allen Frances, I wrote that the APA had an opportunity, using DDPD, to take a leadership role in recognizing as a major problem something that had been largely ignored up to that time. After DDPD was submitted, I never received any communications from Susan Fiester regarding our submission, although DDPD had apparently been assigned to her. I did receive a response to the submission from Allen Frances in a letter dated June 12, 1989, in which he wrote:

> I really wasn't sure what to make about your "delusional dominating personality disorder." How serious are you about it? We intend to be stringent in our requirements for new diagnoses in DSM-IV in a way that I am sure you would endorse. I am very doubtful that "DDPD" has the kind of empirical support necessary for serious inclusion in DSM-IV. [Frances, 1989a, p.1]

On June 23, I wrote to Personality Disorder Chair John Gunderson (with a copy to Frances) to say:

> I submitted [the DDPD proposal] to Allen Frances,

who has just written to ask how seriously we meant
it. The answer ... is "Extremely serious[ly]." Allen
also expressed concern about the empirical base for
the category. I have two answers for this:

(1) It is far, far better than the empirical bases of
many of the categories in the DSM and far, far
better than the empirical bases of some of the categories which (I gather, from talking to the chairs of
the specific DSM groups) apparently will be kept in
the DSM-IV.

(2) There is an abundant empirical base, in all the
work on attitudes toward women, sex differences in
attitudes and beliefs, and so on.

I also said in that letter, "Every group to whom we have
presented this category has responded enthusiastically, recognizing it as a real and heretofore unnamed problem."

On July 24, Frances responded:

As we have discussed, we are taking a very hard line
on new diagnoses for DSM-IV, insisting that they
have extensive empirical support (this includes the
diagnoses in the Appendix that have been of concern to you). We cannot apply the same level of
empirical support to diagnoses already within the
system, especially since there has been insufficient
time for these to be studied systematically and it is
disruptive to constantly tinker with the classification. Thus the argument that a new diagnosis must
meet much higher standards. I also do not give
much weight to enthusiastic endorsements—empirical support is a *sine qua non*. I am enclosing an
article by Blashfield, written independently, which
summarizes some of the reasons for our position.
His requirements are much more stringent than is
possible, but I like the tone. A first step for any new

diagnosis is an empirical review. I don't think that the general literature on attitude towards women provides very pertinent support to the creation of a new diagnosis, but if you are prepared to do the initial work, we will review the material you generate to see if it warrants further consideration and review by the committee.

The above quotation contains a number of interesting points. First, it is not clear what he means when he says that they cannot apply the same stringency to diagnoses already within the system, because there has been insufficient time for them to be studied. This certainly contradicts the claim in the introductory chapter to *DSM-III-R*, that the disorders included in that book are all based on empirical research. In fact, what he seems to be saying is that categories unsupported by valid research will be left in the *DSM* if they are already there.

A second point is that Frances endorses Blashfield's tone but says his requirements are too stringent for the *DSM*; he never does specify what the requirements *ought* to be, how stringent is stringent enough but not too much. This leaves the door wide open to subjectivity and bias.

Third, it is puzzling that he did not consider the research on attitudes toward women to be relevant to DDPD, since many DDPD criteria concern attitudes toward women. At least for the previous revision, the *DSM-III-R* Work Group certainly justified claims about LLPDD's usefulness and validity partly on the basis of research about PMS, which is *not* identical to PMDD. The work group's guidelines about what research is relevant to which categories seem to depend on whether or not they like a particular category.

A fourth issue is that, although Frances said they were

prepared to read the material that we would generate, the only information they gave us about when they would need our review of the relevant work in order to put it through the necessary review was March of 1990; this information came in Gunderson's October 16, 1989, letter to me, after we had made many requests for information about deadlines. Although they told us in October 1989 that they would read a review if they received it by March, a paper they wrote that was published in 1991 makes it clear that they had decided at their October 1989 meeting *not* to give the proposal further consideration.

Fifth, Frances did not deny my remark that DDPD had a stronger scientific foundation than some categories already in the manual but said that that did not matter. He tried to deal with this by claiming that there was not enough time to study existing diagnoses (Is it all right for patients receiving existing, unsupported diagnoses to suffer the harmful consequences?) and by saying that "constantly tinkering with the diagnostic system was disruptive," an astonishing claim from the man who would turn out to be responsible for the most massive set of changes and additions in *DSM* history.

A final point about Frances's letter is related to his comment, after saying we would have to provide empirical support for DDPD, that "If this sounds discouraging, I'm afraid it is meant to." Why should he imagine we would find it discouraging, when that support was precisely what we had told him we planned to gather? It also seems a curious remark from the head of a process that *he* himself claimed was focused *primarily* on amassing and examining empirical data.

At about this time, Frances also wrote to at least one supporter of DDPD to explain that his task force was setting a very high threshold for incorporating any new diagnostic entities, requiring that they have extensive empirical support. While we value your opinion as a clinician and we will take clinical impressions into consideration when reviewing proposed diagnoses, our most important criteria [sic] for inclusion of any category will be its empirical foundation.

As seen in Chapter 4, despite Frances's claim that SDPD would be subjected to equally stringent criteria, the assertion of the primacy of a sound empirical foundation was not borne out.

Gunderson had written to me in August to say that he had arranged for Fiester to review our DDPD proposal, to "be in touch" with me, and to "oversee its discussion at a forthcoming meeting in October." Until after that October meeting was over, no one informed us who would be at the meeting or what would be done there. After the fact, we learned that that was the Personality Disorders Work Group meeting, the minutes of which include no mention whatsoever of DDPD (nor do the minutes from the second of that group's meetings, in March 1990). Gunderson wrote to me: "Like Allen, I would urge you to provide a systematic review of the empirical data supporting your proposal. I also encourage you to consider sex bias issues and how they effect [sic] the available data." After the Personality Disorders Work Group meeting in October, when Gunderson wrote that our SDPD review had arrived too late, he also informed me that he thought it "highly unlikely that enough support [for DDPD] will be available in time for DSM-IV." At that point, he had seen no review of the relevant support and indeed expressed no interest in it—though as I write these words it occurs to me that he might have meant there would be too few backers rather than too little empirical evidence, a meaning that would have been consistent with the political rather than the scientific nature of their process—nor did he claim to have surveyed the relevant literature himself. He then reminded me of the "higher standards" they planned to use for *DSM-IV* and said that "this problem is compounded for a category like DDPD which has neither a widespread clinical tradition nor a significant clinical literature." That is certainly a clear message about the power of tradition, even when it is biased and oppressive. This position was further supported in Gunderson's November 14 letter to me, in which he wrote that "the most formidable obstacle to overcome is the fact that it isn't generally recognized—even if the empirical evidence can be completed." On December 5, Frances had similarly written to me that a major problem with DDPD is that it had no "clinical literature."

Now they had all their doors guarded: Even had we managed the superhuman task of amassing the wealth of relevant data between October and March (while also holding down full-time jobs), the relevant data would not be sufficient because there was no clinical tradition for the category. Surely one has to wonder, when Gunderson says that DDPD is not "generally" recognized, whether he has ever talked to frontline workers at battered wives' shelters, to feminist therapists, and so on. Precisely who constitutes the "general" in their view? Furthermore, as Kutchins and Kirk note, "A new diagnosis, almost by definition, does not have a clinical tradition or literature. In fact, it is often the inclusion of a diagnostic category in *DSM* that allows for a clinical and research tradition to be created to support it."

In what he surely did not mean as ironic, Frances wrote in his October 26 letter to me about DDPD that "it is folly to open the floodgates to new and unsupported diagnoses." No one held the *DSM-III-R* floodgates closed against SDPD and LLPDD, and only opened floodgates could have allowed the increase in number of categories from 297 to the *DSM-IV*'s 374.

In the same letter, Frances implied that I would advocate lower standards for inclusion of our proposed DDPD than for SDPD. On November 8, I wrote to him as follows:

> I certainly don't advocate a different, lower standard for inclusion of DDPD than for any other diagnostic category. In fact, I might have been offended by that implication, but instead I am perplexed. I am all the more perplexed because both you and John Gunderson know that I have offered to put together the empirical materials relevant to DDPD, even though no member of your APA or your DSM Work Group has offered to assist in this, although they do so for other categories. Perhaps you could explain to me why the Work Group's response to our proposal has been consistently discouraging and unsupportive rather than the sort of, "We'll look at the evidence, gather the relevant materials or ask others to help us do that, and then decide" approach that is used for other proposed categories.

In December, Frances sent me another discouraging letter, in which, in Kutchins's and Kirk's view, "there was a rising tone of exasperation with her [Caplan's] efforts and frustration that she would not heed their advice and turn her attention elsewhere."

On February 26, 1990, I wrote to inform Frances that

Fiester had not been in touch with me in regard to DDPD, and on March 5, I wrote to Fiester directly to ask what was happening. I asked her for the names and addresses of other people whom she might have asked to work on DDPD, because "From my work in relation to *DSM-III-R*, I am aware that when new categories are proposed a number of relevant people are asked to work on them. It is important for us to know who these other people are for DDPD." I received no reply to either letter. I had sent Frances copies of those letters, and on March 13, he informed me that he didn't know what the procedure for reviewing DDPD would be and said that that would be Gunderson's responsibility. He added yet again that he was "very much against adding new personality diagnoses and am unaware of any research literature on this newly proposed diagnosis." Candidly, he observed that he "would not recommend that the Work Group devote its resources to this topic as it has more than enough to do already." It would be important to know who decided which of what Frances called the "literally dozens and dozens" of new diagnoses *would* be the beneficiaries of the work group's resources and *how* that was decided. I had also asked Frances how we could apply for some of the research money that the *DSM* Task Force said it was receiving for conducting field trials, because we were interested in conducting a field trial of DDPD. He wrote to me on March 13 to say that they would devote no funds to DDPD and that he did not know what procedure would be used to review our proposal. Write Kutchins and Kirk, "They seemed to have had enough from this woman who did not heed their advice, not recognizing, perhaps, that their advice had been contradictory."

March came and went, and our review of the relevant DDPD research was not yet ready, although a preliminary review of some of that research was ready by July 1990 and was sent to the *DSM* people. The magnitude of the preliminary review of that material showed that there was far too much relevant literature available to have been assembled by March. However, our compilation of relevant, published literature for DDPD was far more massive and substantial than the single-article "data base" available for SDPD at the time that SDPD was voted into the *DSM-III-R!* Furthermore, it reflected the scope and the seriousness of DDPD-related problems. We found that DDPD affects the mental health and well-being of the many men (and some women) who suffer from it, leading to health problems, shortened life spans, problems in relationships, and a reduced capacity for intimacy. They are often plagued by anxiety, stress, homophobia, self-doubt, insecurity, and competitiveness, and they have high rates of drug abuse and violence.

Might the fact that 86 percent of the APA members are male help to explain the work group's welcoming of the misogynist SDPD and avoidance of DDPD? After all, DDPD is implicitly critical of rigid forms of traditional "masculine" socialization. That such an overwhelmingly male association could have a work group that is so unscientific, so lacking in objectivity, however, might surprise those who regard the scientific enterprise as quintessentially male, rational, and objective. Traditionally, mental health practitioners have failed to identify DDPD-type behavior as a problem, because they have equated masculine behavior with normalcy and feminine behavior with pathology. By neglecting to consider extremes of masculine behavior as problematic, we risk the possibility of labeling as SDPD behavior that may be a protective reaction to the damage caused by someone with DDPD. For example, women who "sacrifice [their] own interests for the sake of others" (an SDPD criterion) may do so in an attempt to protect themselves and their children from the abusive behavior of their male partners. As Lenore Walker has pointed out, many of these SDPD types of behavior

> actually appear as part of the normal woman's personality because the sex-role stereotyped patterns teach women to learn to accommodate to the realities of the society as they develop. Rather than self-defeating behaviors . . . in cases where a woman has experienced violence, these behaviors maximize women's chance for survival.

Indeed, the APA seems to have particular trouble with issues of sex, gender, and sexuality. When the *DSM-III-R* was published, the word went out that homosexuality had officially been declared normal, because it was taken out of the *DSM*. Many lesbians and gays were poignantly glad, whether because they believed at some level that the APA actually *knew* what was normal and what was not, or because they were simply relieved to have one official source of pathologizing removed, or some of each. The insidiousness of the *DSM*, however, is reflected in the fact that, contrary to the *DSM* people's public statements about what they had done, homosexuality remained in the manual for some time. A brief summary of the recent history of this issue is that one kind of homosexuality was removed from *DSM-III* but another kind was left in. What went in the manual was "ego dystonic homosexuality," which means that the person did not feel comfortable being homosexual. "Ego syntonic homosexuality," a feeling of virtually complete comfort with being homosexual, was not included. However, in a culture that scorns and demeans lesbians and gay men, it is hard to be completely comfortable with one's homosexuality, and so the *DSM-III* authors were treating as a mental disorder what was often simply a perfectly comprehensible reaction to being mocked and oppressed. To ignore that major social cause of depression, shame, and anguish and instead to mislabel it as individual pathology was irresponsible. In fact, despite the APA's public announcement that homosexuality would not appear in the *DSM-III-R*, a look at its index reveals the listing "Ego dystonic homosexuality," and the instruction "see Sexual Disorders Not Otherwise Specified" on page 296. The listing on page 296 has a five-digit code (302.90), just as all fully approved categories in the main text have, and one kind of sexual disorder listed is "Persistent or marked distress about one's sexual orientation." I could find no listing of homosexuality in *DSM-IV*, although practitioners intent on doing so could choose to list homosexuality under the headings "Sexual Dysfunction Not Otherwise Specified" or "Paraphilias Not Otherwise Specified."

A quite straightforward gender bias aspect of what we might call *DSM*gate was the *DSM* authors' claim that they rejected DDPD because it targeted a specific group (men, I assume, although we had specified that women could also fit the description), but SDPD (mostly) and LLPDD (entirely) target one specific population, that is, women, and the authors were eager to include both of those categories in the manual.

Apart from biases about gender, it is also possible that the APA's resistance to considering DDPD was because, by proposing the category, we implicitly raised fundamental questions about their whole definition of "mental disorder." Certainly, one cannot read the criteria for DDPD without wondering how "mental disorder" ought to be defined, and this may simply have been an enterprise the *DSM* people did not wish to take on.

Many of the task force's biases are obvious, some more blatant than others. Occasionally, they drop all pretense of fairness. In April 1986 I was preparing a chapter for *The Myth of Women's Masochism* about the revisions process for the *DSM-III-R*. I telephoned Steve Sharfstein, then deputy medical director of the APA, to ask him to verify some quotations that I recalled from the Ad Hoc Committee's December 1985 hearings on the controversial categories. I told Sharfstein (April 15, 1986) that I remembered that the proceedings had been tape-recorded and wondered if I could have a copy of the tapes or a transcript. I explained that I wanted to avoid misquoting anyone. He told me that I could not have access to that information, and his words were so striking that I wrote them down at the time: "This is not the government," he said. "There's no freedom of information here."

In April 1991, an article I had written containing much of the story in this chapter and the previous one was published under the title "How *Do* They Decide Who Is Normal?" in the journal *Canadian Psychology/Psychologie Canadienne*. When its editor, Patrick O'Neill, had asked me who might write a reply to my paper, I said I thought that Allen Frances and his colleagues should be given a chance to respond. He extended that invitation, and Frances responded in a two-and-a-half-page article he coauthored with no fewer than six other people (the first three listed after his name were men with M.D. and Ph.D. degrees, and the three listed as the last coauthors were all women with master's degrees). In their article, they simply asserted that the process of the *DSM* revisions task force was not political but rather was "a careful three-stage process of empirical review and documentation which strives as much as is possible to base decisions on data rather than expert opinion and argument." (See Chapter 7 for further elaboration about this issue.) They also said that summaries of the information *at each stage of the process* were "widely distributed to critics (including Dr. Caplan)." Although they may have been widely distributed, if their dealings with me were typical of their dealings with critics, they did *not* circulate summaries at all three stages, nor did they make it possible to provide feedback in time for the deadlines they set, nor did they take the feedback into account when it did not further their aims. I am also informed that they did not even consult with some of the professionals—such as representatives of the American Psychological Association—whom they had promised to use as advisors.

In their paper, Frances and his colleagues accused me of feeling that they "should come to closure on the issues she is concerned with far earlier than is necessary or appropriate." This is an interesting claim in view of the breathtaking prematurity of many of their decisions, such as about SDPD for *DSM-III-R* and PMDD for *DSM-IV*.

They used their article to advertise some of the big moneymaking publications that would be produced around the same time as the *DSM-IV*, such as the *DSM-IV Source Book*. They also said they planned to produce a DSM-IV Options Book that would be "distributed widely to the field," so that people could see the various possibilities that were under consideration before the handbook's contents were finalized. This gave the impression that they were open to thoughtful suggestions. However, some of the best options, such as Judith Gold's proposal to list LLPDD simply under the category of "Medical Conditions," were ignored, while a less scientific and more irresponsible method of choosing a recommendation was selected.

Editor O'Neill gave me the chance to reply to the response article by Frances et al., and I called my brief answer "Response to the DSM Wizard," pointing out the parallel between the behavior of Frances and his colleagues and that of the man who pretended to be a wizard in *The Wizard of Oz*. In the film about Oz, when Toto the dog pulls back a curtain and reveals that what is supposed to be a wizard with magical powers is just a man cranking a machine, the pretender looks at Dorothy and her friends and tries to convince them that the truth is not what they think they are seeing.

In their article, Frances et al. repeatedly used the word *consensus*: some of their allegedly empirically based decisions, they acknowledged, would be based, as before, on consensus. However, the consensus to which they referred came from their handful of colleagues, as described. In view of the strong objections to some of the *DSM-IV* categories that have come from all quarters, the *DSM-IV* authors' claim to work by any kind of broadly based consensus seems absurd.

7

How Gatekeeping Replaces Scientific Precision

DSM-III represents a bold series of choices based on guess, taste, prejudice, and hope ... few are based on fact or truth.
— George Vaillant, "A Debate on DSM-III"

In the world of modern psychiatry, claims can become truth, hopes can become achievements, and propaganda is taken as science.
— Peter Breggin, *Toxic Psychiatry*

My observations of the *DSM* process have taught me that far too little science goes into producing the handbook.* Far more than being based on careful research, the handbook's contents are determined by the powerful *DSM* leaders' gatekeeping—unscientific decisions about which diagnoses will be allowed through and which will be kept out of the handbook. To the untutored eye, and even to many mental health personnel, the *DSM* appears grounded in science, although many features that give this impression turn out on inspection to provide only

---

*Portions of this chapter were taken from Paula J. Caplan, Afterword: A warning. *The myth of women's masochism* (New York: Signet, 1987); from June Larkin and Paula J.Caplan, The gatekeeping process of the *DSM*. *Canadian Journal of Community Mental Health* 11 (1992):17–28; and from Kaye-Lee Pantony and Paula J. Caplan, Science vs. conjecture in the *DSM* (1993, unpublished paper).

a veneer of scientific sheen rather than genuine, carefully supported research. Many people assume that, with all the developments in science and the burgeoning of mental health systems, surely decisions about who is normal are scientifically and responsibly made. But the excellence of science/technology in designing airplanes does not guarantee excellence and precision in diagnosis. After all, a plane either flies or it doesn't, but many of the consequences of diagnosis and misdiagnosis are less clear.

At first glance, the *DSM* is impressive: In addition to its physical size, it includes a huge list of names of professionals who are said to have contributed to the manual's development; in the *DSM-IV*, the acknowledgments section begins with the words, "DSM-IV is a team effort. More than 1000 people and numerous professional organizations have helped us in the preparation of this document." In fact, they do include a list of more than a thousand names at the back of the book, but the vast majority are white male American psychiatrists, and I know that the list includes many names of people whose work was not incorporated into their decision-making. Furthermore, the core players are task force and work group members, but of those whose sex could be identified from their names, twenty-five members of the task force were male but only five were female (and the women were primarily described as "coordinator," "administrative assistant," and so on, rather than as holding the more powerful and high-status roles). Of those work group members whose sex was clear from their names, eighty were men but only fifteen were women (and this includes the six-member all-woman LLPDD Work Group).

The fact that the manual is known to be undergoing constant revision contributes to the impression that science is involved and that new, high-quality studies must impel these revisions. The *DSM* authors' repeated references to their "field trial" research—which is supposed to be composed of studies of the handbook's use in actual clinical practice—also make the process sound scientific. Their production of a report of their research in the *DSM-IV Sourcebook*, in no less than five volumes, is, they say, "intended to provide a comprehensive and convenient reference record of the clinical and research support for the various decisions reached."

The APA's own publication about *DSM-IV*, called *Fact Sheet*, strongly contributes to the impression that the manual is based on sound scientific research that leads clearly to effective treatment:

> Psychiatrists depend on accurate diagnostic tools to help them identify precisely the mental illnesses their patients suffer, an essential step in deciding what treatment or combination of treatments the patient needs. . . . *DSM-IV* is based on decades of research and the input of thousands of psychiatric experts from across the country and in every subspecialty. . . . *DSM-IV* has been carefully written and exhaustively researched. . . .
>
> As research has increased psychiatry's understanding of mental illnesses and sharpened its ability to diagnose and treat them, the *DSM* has changed to reflect this greater level of sophistication. . . .
>
> According to Dr. Allen Frances, Chair of the *DSM-IV* Task Force, "The major innovation of *DSM-IV* lies not in any of its specific content changes, but rather in the systematic and explicit process by which it was constructed and documented. More than any other nomenclature of mental disorders, *DSM-IV* is grounded in empirical evidence."

... The Task Force set high standards for evaluating proposals for changes in the new manual. Recommended changes had to be substantiated by explicit statements of rationale, supported by the systematic review of relevant empirical data.

In *DSM-IV*, 374 different kinds of mental disorder are listed under categories, subcategories, and sub-subcategories, with information for each diagnosis about associated features and disorders; specific age, cultural, or gender-related features; prevalence, incidence, and risk; course; complications; predisposing factors; familial pattern; and differential diagnosis. This certainly makes it appear as though research must be available to reveal all of that information for every category, but that is not the case. Each category and subcategory is given a multidigit number including a period, which suggests that the manual enables one to make extremely fine distinctions among disorders, as between 307.46 and 307.47. Each category has a label and a long list of highly specific criteria for that category, giving the impression that someone has found out for sure that that kind of mental disorder is characterized by those criteria. Each category has a cutoff point, such as that the patient must meet five of the nine criteria listed in order to be assigned that particular label; this makes it seem as though research has been carefully done to determine that, for instance, people regarded as having Major Depressive Episode do indeed meet five of the nine criteria listed under that label and that people who meet four or fewer do not suffer from that disorder. In the introduction to *DSM-IV* one can find a couple of sentences indicating that one should use one's clinical judgment about the number of criteria the patient needs to meet, but it is probably safe to say that few people read every word of the introduction and still fewer remember its contents. Furthermore, if one is supposed to use one's clinical judgment in applying these categories, then science goes out the window, for one of the claims most loudly and frequently made about the *DSM* by its authors is that it ensures that research will be properly done, with everyone defining, for instance, "Major Depressive Episode" identically. The most useful kind of research is done on real patients in real treatment settings, the very places where "clinical judgment" in the form of deviations from the *DSM* criteria's rules are most likely to be made; this means that the best places to do potentially useful research are the places where controlled science is least likely to be done.

What perhaps contributes most to the *DSM*'s aura of scientific precision is simply its authors' repeated allegations that it is scientifically grounded. The second sentence of the introduction to *DSM-IV* reads: "The utility and credibility of DSM-IV require that it focus upon its clinical, research and educational purposes and be supported by an extensive empirical foundation." The authors go on to say that twelve field trials were conducted at more than seventy sites, including more than six thousand patients, and that "The field trials collected information on the reliability and performance characteristics of each criteria set as a whole as well as of the specific items within each criteria set."

It has been fascinating to observe the historical process of the *DSM* authors of each successive edition claiming that whichever edition was then being prepared would be different from the previous ones in that *this* new one would be truly scientifically grounded. The *DSM-III-R* chiefs said that their edition would be a vast improvement over the unscientific *DSM-III*. Spitzer said that the solid empirical basis of *DSM-III-R* not only would distinguish it from *III* but was *the* most compelling reason to produce a *III-R*. And in a 1991 article, Allen Frances and his coauthors claimed, "The major difference between the preparation of DSM-IV and that of DSM-III and III-R is its emphasis on explicit review and documentation of the available data." Were the consequences for millions of people not so devastating, the predictable reappearances of these claims would be as funny as a repeated gag in a Marx Brothers movie.

The belief that the handbook is scientifically grounded does not remain confined to its authors but spreads to the wider community. In *The New Psychiatrists*, a book written for laypeople, Jerrold Maxmen made the unqualified announcement that "On July 1, 1980, the ascendance of scientific psychiatry became official. For on this day, the APA published a radically different system for psychiatric diagnosis called . . . DSM-III"—and then he asserted that American psychiatrists had adopted "the scientifically based DSM-III as its official system for diagnosis." He also claimed, "Scientific psychiatry bases truth on scientific experimentation. . . . The old psychiatry derives from theory, the new psychiatry from fact."

Why do we need to worry about whether or not the *DSM* is scientifically sound? After all, during twenty-five years in the field of psychology, I have found that most of the truly fine therapists say that when they are able to be of use to people who come to them for help, what works isn't easy to measure. Sometimes, it is not even easy to identify, because it has to do primarily with the nature of the relationship between therapist and patient, the degree of trust, empathy, sense of humor, intelligence of certain kinds, and so on. But the question of scientific validity is key in regard to the *DSM* because, if the *DSM-*

related science is unsound, the stated aims for the *DSM* and many of the book's actual uses are at least absurd, if not outright harmful. Of course, even if the science were sound, labels can still be misused.

A deeply disturbing consequence of the *DSM*'s lack of science is that reasonably intelligent people assume that labels in the handbook correspond to disorders or problems that are known to exist. When categories are presented as though they are real, it is inevitable that some people will be classified as belonging to those categories and will be given various treatments aimed to cure their supposed mental disorders. For nonexistent disorders, this is a waste of time, energy, and money if the patient is lucky, and it is profoundly harmful if the patient is less fortunate. Putting a leg in a cast for a patient who has in fact broken her arm—or who only has a sprained ankle—is harmful; so, too, is calling a woman premenstrually mentally ill when she is only feeling as angry or sad as many women and men do much of the time, or when she is depressed because she lost her job or has a sick child. Similarly, calling an abused person or a target of racism self-defeating does them significant harm. The authors of that first poor empirical study of "Masochistic Personality Disorder" had reported that one characteristic of people with that alleged disorder was that they had a "negative therapeutic reaction," which means that they got worse after becoming psychotherapy patients. Kass and his colleagues presented this important bit of information without attempting to explain it. Most likely, they assumed it was simply another manifestation of the patients' masochism, their presumed wish to avoid feeling better. However, as I learned from people who had been the patients of therapists who believed in this disorder, those "negative therapeutic reactions" are virtually inevitable results of

being told that one has a deep-seated need to feel miserable, that one brings all one's troubles on oneself, that there
is no point in leaving a bad situation because one's unconscious masochism will just drive one out in search of another one that is at least as bad.

The mistaken assumption that the *DSM* is scientifically
sound has led to confusion on the part of clinicians and
to heartache on the part of patients and their families.
Suppose that, like a couple with whom I consulted some
years ago, you have a five-year-old son who barely speaks,
who cannot do many of the things most five-year-olds do,
but who is warm and loving and seems reasonably happy.
You desperately want to help your son to continue to live
a happy life, but you know there is a lot of trouble in
store for him as he gets older and as the disparity between
what he and his age-mates can do continues to grow. You
seek help from various pediatricians, psychiatrists, and ed-
ucators. None has ever seen a child like yours, and as
you progress through the consultations, various labels are
proposed for him. Some say he is mentally retarded, others
say he is severely learning disabled or developmentally disabled or minimally brain-damaged, and still others say that
he is autistic. Depending on which label sticks, very different kinds of treatments will be suggested for him. If he is
considered profoundly retarded, some people will tell you
he should be placed in a residential setting with other,
equally slow children so that he won't feel so out of his
depth. This will mean a dramatic and quite possibly traumatic separation from you. If he has a number of severe
learning disabilities, then an intensive program of remedi-
ation may be suggested by some professionals, perhaps
with one set of exercises for his speech delay, another set
for his trouble in using scissors, still another for his inability to climb stairs without tripping, and so on. If he is

classified as autistic, some professionals will recommend institutionalizing him, some will tell you that you (especially the mother) should be more affectionate toward him, some will say he should be put on a strict behavior modification program to teach him each of the skills he lacks, and some will prescribe drugs of different kinds for him.

Not only the recommendations but also the prognoses you will be offered will vary a great deal, depending on which label he is given. "Severe mental retardation" is not generally believed to change very much. "Developmental delays" and "learning disabilities" are widely considered to be problems that many people outgrow over time. "Autism" usually makes people's hearts sink with a sense of hopelessness, although a few professionals have claimed to be able to help these children considerably or even "cure" them.

The couple who brought their five-year-old to see me had spent a great deal of time inspecting the description of "Infantile Autism" in the *DSM*. It was terribly important to them to figure out whether or not he was autistic, they said, because they wanted to tailor their expectations to meet what he was likely to be able to do. Furthermore, they knew that the kinds of treatments that professionals would use might depend in part on his diagnosis. The parents' aims were perfectly reasonable and caring, but the way they sought answers to their questions was based on the belief that there was clearly such a phenomenon as "Infantile Autism" and that it would be possible to determine definitively whether or not their son belonged in that category. Even those of us who work in the mental health professions often act as though we believe there is some absolute reality to most categories of mental disorders. But as noted, *all* mental disorders listed in the *DSM* are constructs. If they were not, the process would be to find people who are, for instance, autistic, write down their characteristics, and then use the handbook very much like a guide to South American birds: if it has yellow wings and a blunt, black bill, it must be Bird X. But because we depend so much on the powers of observation (what we look at, how accurate our observations are, how consistent our observations are of one person compared to another) and on the mythical uniformity of human beings, it is not like that for mental disorders. We are not content simply to look at people as individuals and think carefully and humanely about what might help them; we insist on classifying them. This makes enormous sense to me, in principle. After all, if I knew that, *if* that little boy met all six of the criteria listed under "Infantile Autism" in the *DSM*, a certain kind of medication or assistance would help him, I'd be delighted to stick the label on him. Or even if applying the label enabled me to tell his parents that he probably would never learn to read or speak, I would at least be glad I could give them a chance to prepare for the likely future of their son. But despite the fact that massive amounts of writing about "Infantile Autism" have been done, no one has ever produced the kinds of data that would make it clear that this is a condition that can be unambiguously defined, that any particular person can be shown for certain to "have" or "not have" it (see later in this chapter).

It was heartbreaking to see the five-year-old boy's parents searching desperately for a label that would fit him rather than exploring what possible treatments—for autism or anything else—might help him. It was not surprising that they might assume that finding the right label would tell them what would help. These parents were understandably reluctant to try any treatment unless they knew it had been helpful for other children who had been given a label that seemed to fit their child. Unfortunately, their reluctance grew out of the mistaken belief that ample, responsible, scientific work had been done, work that had led to discoveries of likely improvements or cures from certain treatments applied to children who had been given particular labels.

The *DSM* authors diverge from responsible scientific practice, as I shall now describe, by designing and conducting studies in sloppy ways, by distorting their findings to make them look better than they are, and by not revealing some of their findings or revealing them too late to give non-*DSM* people time to respond before the next edition of the handbook is published. Another serious problem is that some *DSM* research was conducted at sites supervised by or employing *DSM* committee members, whose stake in the *DSM*'s success might well have affected the ways they did their part of the study. Based on decades of research on "experimenter bias," people who want a particular category included in the manual might make mistakes in collecting and reporting data that would tend to make that category look more reliable than it actually is.

When I was serving as a member of the two work groups for the *DSM-IV*, I clung absurdly long to the assumption that Fiester's and Gold's slowness, or failure, in sending us materials and information must have been oversights due to their being overworked, but when I read Kirk and Kutchins's book *The Selling of DSM*, I realized that this was standard conduct in the *DSM* project. As Kirk and Kutchins comment, "No full, comprehensive report with methodological details [of the research about the handbook] was ever made available."

The studies conducted for the manual are of two kinds:

evaluations of the *content* of diagnostic categories—whether the criteria for a category accurately and adequately describe that "disorder"—and *reliability* checks to see whether two different therapists will assign the same label to the same patient. Robert Spitzer has said that the content evaluations for his *DSM-III* and *DSM-III-R* were used to revise the criteria for various categories. This research involved asking psychiatrists which criteria for a given category they found useful, whether they had other criteria to suggest, and so on—all very subjective questions. There is nothing wrong with trying to gather information by such polls, but it is not scientific in and of itself. Although many people may believe that a certain "disorder" is characterized by a particular problem, they may all be mistaken in that belief. Therefore, careful research needs to be done to determine whether, for instance, all children who have "Autistic Disorder" actually have language problems. Of course, this is where the kinds of problems discussed in relation to all constructs arise. Until and unless some infallible test is discovered for something that is called a mental disorder, there is no way to "find out" what "Autistic Disorder," for instance, *really is*. All one could do would be to approach those who seem to know the most about "Autistic Disorder," keeping in mind that it may not exist as such, then ask those people what they think its characteristics are, compile a list of characteristics on that basis, and find out whether thousands of children who have been diagnosed (but by whom? the acknowledged experts? the average clinician?) as "Autistic" actually meet those criteria. (As we shall see later in this chapter, the *DSM* architects did not do this.) Of course, if many such children do not meet those criteria, that may be because there is no such real phenomenon as "Autistic Disorder," or it could mean that several different kinds of problems are lumped together under that label, or that there is such a phenomenon but some therapists are better than others at recognizing it. So what Spitzer and his colleagues did in order to choose criteria for their categories in one sense was not terribly wrong but is not conclusive proof that those categories are valid. Their method, which so often consists of chatting with or surveying chosen colleagues, looking at some research but not basing many decisions on what it tells them, and then handing down fiats, cannot be considered particularly sound. And in a sense what they did was deeply wrong because of the lack of diversity among the people providing input and making the final choices (mostly white male North American psychiatrists), for the less diversity one has in these kinds of subjective endeavors, the more likely biases are to go uncorrected by people who, belonging to different groups, might be likely to bring fresh perspectives to the *DSM* project.

As mentioned, some of the research on the *DSM* editions that has been cited as "proof" of the manual's scientific foundation has never even been published. Almost all of the research that *has* been published is about inter-rater reliability—whether two therapists will assign the same patient the same diagnosis—and even that is of very poor quality. Reliability is certainly crucial, but even if the handbook produced terrific reliability data, much would be lacking, for reliability information tells us nothing at all about whether the labels they are assigning have any *validity*, any reality. After all, one could get a large group of people to agree to call all horses "unicorns," so that their inter-rater reliability would be perfect, but that would not mean that any of them ever really saw unicorns.

Kirk and Kutchins have traced the way that, beginning with the *DSM-III*, the authors have managed to create the unjustified impression that reliability problems have largely been solved. Their public relations has been so skilled that it has been widely assumed that the major hurdle in achieving good inter-rater reliability was overcome in the *DSM-III* and that subsequent reliability research has been about minor details. In fact, though, their own research reveals that *DSM-III* and *III-R* improved either very little or not at all on the reliability of diagnostic categories from earlier editions. That simple fact has been lost in the morass of claims by Spitzer and his colleagues about the good reliability of their categories. Frankly, few therapists of any kind take the trouble to read the papers about the handbook's reliability in which the actual data— which by all rights should embarrass the *DSM* authors—are presented. As a result, the authors' claims about improved reliability are rarely questioned. As noted, much of the research to which Spitzer and his colleagues refer has never been published and hence is not available for inspection by those who might question their claims to scientific validity. (Even as an advisor to a *DSM* work group, I was not given access to much of the unpublished data; see Chapter 4.) But I was able to locate three publications, including the *DSM-III* itself, in which the research on the reliability of the *DSM-III* was reported, and because so little work has been done since then, it is worth looking briefly at what those revealed.

Spitzer, Forman, and Nee explored whether two different psychiatrists would assign the same diagnostic label to the same patient. For some cases, the two psychiatrists saw the same patient simultaneously, and for others, the patient was seen at different times by each. The authors claimed that this study showed that "reliability is quite good," but in fact under the second circumstance, which most closely approximates what happens in real clinical practice, the reliability was poor. Clinicians were asked to assign what the *DSM* lists as Axis I and Axis II labels. Axis II disorders consist of Personality Disorders (generally defined as a maladaptive organization of one's entire personality, such as Paranoid Personality) and Specific Developmental Disorders (such as Developmental Arithmetic Disorder). Axis I includes all other mental disorders. When two therapists saw the same patient at different times, they agreed only about half of the time (actually, 54 percent of the time, which is usually written by researchers as .54) for Axis II disorders and only about two thirds of the time (.66) for Axis I disorders. For therapists, who have spent years in expensive training programs, to diverge so dramatically when using the *DSM* does not say much for the *DSM* category descriptions. Even when the therapists observed the same patient *at the same time*, they agreed just over half of the time (.61) for Axis II and a little more than three-fourths of the time (.78) for Axis I disorders. Now, the .78 figure might seem pretty good if one did not know two crucial facts about the study. One is that for seven of the twenty-five diagnostic categories, the inter-rater agreement was 1.00—agreement about every patient—figures that did a great deal to raise the overall averages to .78 and .61 in the simultaneous interviews; but those seven categories included, respectively, only two, five, one, one, three, one, and three patients. It is not particularly impressive that two therapists could agree about whether or not one or a very few cases would be classified the same. Furthermore, the next highest inter-rater reliability figure was .90, and that was for thirty-three patients diagnosed as having Substance Use Disorders— obviously an easy category to identify.

The whole rationale for expanding *DSM* from a handful of briefly named categories to hundreds of lengthilydescribed categories and subcategories was that greater scientific precision would result from the latter. However, the already unimpressive statistics just given apply only to therapists' decisions about which of a few *major* categories, not subcategories, to apply to patients. The entire study could have been done with the far more terse *DSM-II*. I would not be surprised if laypeople could do as well as the therapists in this study, for it does not take much to decide whether someone is alcoholic in contrast to manic, for instance. What would have been impressive would have been to achieve good inter-rater reliability for therapists trying to decide whether a particular patient "has," for instance, Generalized Anxiety Disorder in contrast to Atypical Anxiety Disorder.

In a second study, Hyler, Williams, and Spitzer compared therapists' choice of diagnoses for patients they had seen in interviews to their choice for patients about whom they had only read in case summaries. They found higher reliability between raters using interviews than case summaries, but again, they reported only the data for agreement about the major diagnostic categories, not the subcategories. One can only imagine how low the reliability figures on the latter must have been. The overall degree of agreement between raters was only .67, so that they agreed only about two-thirds of the time, and as with the previous study, this was artificially elevated by three categories (out of a total of sixteen) that included only one patient each, one that included only three patients, and the .95 level for a handful of the hard-to-misdiagnose Substance Use Disorder label.

In the *DSM-III* itself, the reliability material appears either to be the same as those from the studies just reported or to overlap a great deal with them, and the figures and problems with them are similar. Despite the fact that their own research showed their new classification system to have poor reliability, the very listing of tables and charts with many numbers can give the impression of great scientific precision and significant scientific achievement. (Kirk and Kutchins describe the ways Spitzer and his colleagues reported different figures and research procedures at different times, calling into further question the seriousness with which one should take their claims.)

On the basis of such pitiful results did Spitzer often make such pronouncements as that the reliability of *III* was "quite good, and in general it was much higher than that previously achieved with DSM-I and DSM-II," although that was not true. Spitzer and his colleagues first chose a fairly high number for their standard of "good reliability" but lowered it to .70 when their data began to come in. Even so, based on their own reports of the *DSM-III* research, of the eighty mental disorders in adults for which they reported results, inter-rater reliabilities for only thirty-one categories were above .70, while forty-nine were below. For the twenty-four disorders in childhood and adolescence for which they gave figures, only eight were above the .70 level, and four of those eight had reliabilities of 1.00 but were based on only *one* patient each! As with the research on SDPD, these studies could go in a textbook as examples of poorly executed and irresponsibly interpreted research. Kirk and Kutchins summarize the *DSM-III* research by saying:

> The field trials themselves could more accurately be described as uncontrolled, nonrandom surveys in which several hundred self-selected and unsupervised pairs of clinicians throughout the country at-

tempted to diagnose nonrandomly selected patients and, after some sharing of information, made "independent" assessments of these patients. . . .

One of the legacies of the DSM-III field trials, described as the largest field trials in psychiatric history, is how little is actually known about such an ostensibly important study. No book was written, no complete technical report was made available to other researchers, no final summary report was produced, and the data set was not made available for reanalysis by other investigators.

In 1984, Gerald Klerman, "the highest-ranking psychiatrist in the federal government" when *DSM-III* was adopted, had the temerity to announce that the problem of reliability had been solved by the *DSM-III* and that the handbook embodied "science in the service of healing . . . to a greater extent than any other achievement in American psychiatry since the advent of the new drugs." However, an investigation that was conducted first before and then two years after *III* was published showed that the new *DSM* had affected assignment of diagnoses very little.

When it came time for *DSM-III-R*, Spitzer and his colleagues must have felt they could pretty much relax about reliability, for they did even less work than before on it, focused on a few disorders, obtained low response rates from the people they asked to participate in their research, and only published some of their results in journals many years later. Some of their work apparently never has been published, and in *DSM-III-R*, the authors did not even bother to report what they had found, and they got away with not mentioning it. Whereas the field trials for *III* apparently included most or all of the major categories in the manual, according to the manual itself, those for *III-R* included only *seven* categories out of the nearly three hundred that are listed in that edition. Of the seven, five are disorders found in children (Attention-Deficit Hyperactivity Disorder, Oppositional Defiant Disorder, Conduct Disorder, Autistic Disorder, and Pervasive Developmental Disorder), and two are found mostly in adults (Agoraphobia Without History of Panic Disorder and Generalized Anxiety Disorder). Not only do the *III-R* authors not report any of the field trials' results whatsoever but they do not even say in the manual where one might go to find these numbers.

Although no reliability studies are mentioned in *III-R*, I located a study published in 1992, which was coauthored by Janet Williams, Robert Spitzer, and no less than nine other people. For the 390 "mental patients" they studied, therapists' agreement about diagnoses was below the .70 level for forty-three categories, and only seventeen were above that level. The higher figures came for such easy-to-call labels as bulimia and alcohol and drug dependence. All in all, this study was a very poor showing by those who wished to claim high reliability for that edition of the manual.

In brief, the research shows that *DSM* reliability is poor, that two therapists are not impressively likely to assign the same label (even for broad, not highly specific, categories) to the same person. A cardinal rule of reliability research is that if inter-rater agreement is not good, we cannot begin to assume that the categories represent anything real. The analogy used by researchers Mirowsky and Ross is an apt one: When different people look up at the stars, there are, in fact, no "real" constellations; rather, people agree to divide up the heavens into certain groupings of stars rather than making the division some other way, and then they agree to call one group the Big Dipper, another Orion, and so on. This is similar to two therapists dividing up an array of patients into categories in different ways, which is what inter-rater reliability is all about.

For *DSM-IV*, an official APA publication, "Fact Sheet" (which title I assume they do not intend to be ironic), presents *IV* as "exhaustively researched." The unnamed writer of that sheet claims that the *DSM-IV* is organized "by groups of symptoms which are commonly associated with a specific illness," thus clearly identifying mental problems with "illnesses" and also implying a scientific foundation that could reveal the "association" of certain symptoms with a particular "illness." That writer then claims that a "three-stage empirical review" was carried out, beginning with 150 reviews of the scientific literature on which decisions about *IV* would be based. My own experience with the poor quality and/or the misrepresentation of the data in reports by *DSM-IV* work group personnel about the existing research for SDPD and LLPDD makes me wince when I read their claims about their literature reviews. The "Fact Sheet" writer next mentions twelve field trials, giving the information that they were funded by the National Institute of Mental Health, National Institute on Drug Abuse, and National Institution of Alcoholism and Alcohol Abuse but saying nothing about how the field trials were designed or executed or how the information from those trials was analyzed. This is unforgivable in the realm of scientific methodology.

Summarizing the alleged findings from this research, the APA's Harold Pincus, vice-chairperson of the *DSM-IV* Task Force and director of APA's Office of Research, claimed in the "Fact Sheet," "The process of systematically examining the empirical data has enabled us to reach remarkable consensus on the literally hundreds of decisions made by the Task Force." Sounds very scientific indeed, but when I read the word *consensus*, I recall from my own experiences with their work groups what they describe as "consensus." It is easy enough for them to claim that all of this was done in an "open process" if they are never called on to prove it.

The "science" related to the *DSM-III, III-R,* and *IV* overall, then, is inadequate and of poor quality. However, most of that research is about inter-rater reliability, and in theory one might obtain such poor reliability if one had scientifically well-validated categories of mental disorders but if therapists' diagnostic skills were bad. Therefore, it is important also to consider the "science" related to the validity of some specific categories: What is the evidence that they refer to real phenomena and that they describe them accurately? The sparse and shoddy research related to SDPD and LLPDD has been mentioned in Chapters 4 and 5 but warrants some further description here. According to Lenore Walker, the criteria for SDPD were "originally . . . created by two of the male members on the task force in a rowboat while waiting for the fish to bite." Remember that the APA voted to introduce SDPD into the *DSM* at a time when only a single piece of empirical research related to it was in existence, and that piece of research was a model of poor science. As noted, all it really showed was that a few Columbia University Psychiatry Department psychiatrists (who probably knew that one of the researchers was heading the *DSM-III-R* group and was a staunch supporter of "Masochistic Personality Disorder") consistently applied the term "masochistic personality" to a group of traits that were chosen from very old anecdotal papers. This does not prove that there is such a thing as a masochistic personality; it only proves that people working in the same setting may give the same label—rightly or wrongly—to a set of behavior descriptions. If we decide to call all horses zebras, the animals do not break out in stripes. There were eight more major methodological errors, including the fact that only fifty-nine patients were studied, a very small number in any case and especially in view of the fact that Spitzer and his colleagues claimed that only a small percentage of any population of patients would receive the "Masochistic" diagnosis.

At nearly the last minute before *DSM-III-R* was to be approved, Spitzer made another misguided attempt to create a research base to support SDPD. In January 1986 he sent out a letter cosigned by Frederic Kass and Janet Williams, on APA letterhead stationery, although there was nothing else to suggest that this was a project of the APA itself rather than of a few members of one of its groups. Their letter was accompanied by a questionnaire designed "to obtain data that will help determine how many of the eight diagnostic criteria are necessary to make the diagnosis." Thus, a category that had not yet been approved by the APA Board for inclusion in the handbook acquired respectability by being the subject of a study announced on official Association stationery. Furthermore, as the above wording makes clear, the category was presented as though the diagnosis were a sure thing and the only question was exactly what the cutoff point for the criteria should be. This is not the way that such a questionnaire should ever have been worded. If there were such a thing as SDPD, then researchers should set out to find people who clearly have SDPD ("clearly" usually meaning that some respected therapists believe these people have SDPD) and study how many of the criteria most or all of them meet. Spitzer and his colleagues were basically asking some members of APA to cast a vote about what the cutoff point should be. Imagine asking a bunch of orthopedic surgeons to vote on how many symptoms of a broken rib have to be present in order to prove that a patient has a broken rib, rather than studying correlations between X rays of ribs and records of symptoms of patients whose ribs do and patients whose ribs do not turn out to be broken.

Psychiatrist Marjorie Braude received the questionnaire, and she pointed out that it was constructed in a way that guaranteed dramatically skewed responses: "The questionnaire . . . asks if I believe that the diagnosis of self-defeating personality disorder should be included in the revised DSM-III. . . . If I answer yes I am asked to go on to describe characteristics of specific cases. If I answer no I simply return the questionnaire without any clinical data. By including only data from psychiatrists who think there is a need for the diagnosis one will obtain skewed . . . results." A bizarre note is that, in reply to such criticism, Spitzer reported that about half of the people who returned their questionnaires said they did *not* believe the category should be included in *DSM-III-R*. In view of this, how he could proceed with the diagnosis is difficult to comprehend. Kutchins and Kirk report that only 31 percent of the questionnaire recipients returned it, and only about one-third of those completed the instructions, so that the data "are based on only 11 percent of the sample, a small subgroup of respondents who had been deliberately screened into the study by the researchers and who, we can assume, were among those most supportive of the proposal for SDPD." Even so, this piece of research revealed that each of the traits listed for SDPD was present in between 29 percent and 51 percent of the patients who were *not* thought to have SDPD, clearly showing that SDPD is not a discrete entity.

As the reviews done by Wendy Schwartz, Judith Herman, and Maureen Gans and myself have shown, the few additional pieces of research on SDPD that appeared between 1986 and the time that *DSM-IV* was being prepared continued to fail to support the claim that there even is such a phenomenon as SDPD. Like earlier studies, the new work was deeply flawed and also reinforced our earlier concern that powerful gender biases were at work in the way the label was applied. As noted, Susan Fiester, the psychiatrist heading the SDPD subcommittee, wrote her own review of the literature, but it included contradictions and errors of fact in reporting what had been found in various studies, and the logic in her summary of the research was faulty. For instance, she cited studies that had been extensively discredited methodologically as though they had not been. She also mentioned a study that actually provided evidence that SDPD was not a legitimate construct but did not say that that was what it showed. She lumped together with SDPD criteria those criteria that had been part of "Masochistic Personality Disorder" but had not made it into the list for "Self-Defeating Personality Disorder," but her paper was to be used to decide whether or not SDPD should stay in the manual. As I wrote in my critique of Fiester's review, lumping these studies together was "like adding together slightly rotten apples and terribly rotten apples and claiming one comes up with a sum total of fresh apples."

The Personality Disorders Work Group sent me a copy of the minutes from their September 19–20, 1991, meeting, which shows that at that point—before the publicity in Dr. Margaret Jensvold's sex discrimination case against the National Institute of Mental Health—they decided to recommend officially that SDPD be retained in the appendix. This apparently was done in spite of their claim that they required strong scientific support for their categories. They certainly seemed to be putting into practice Allen Frances's statement that his group would use lower scientific standards for diagnoses that were already in the manual than for proposals for new ones. But this also shows that they did not take seriously the label they gave to the appendix in which SDPD appears, that of a *provisional appendix for categories needing further study*. Just imagine: You can get your favorite category into the *DSM* appendix with no decent scientific research to back it up by claiming that that doesn't matter, since the appendix is for provisional categories. Then, once it has appeared in that appendix, you get to keep it in the manual even though there is still no good supporting research for it, on the grounds that, according to Frances, one cannot run around making major changes to existing categories, because it plays havoc with clinical practice and research. That is precisely what the *DSM* authors have done with SDPD and LLPDD.

In regard to LLPDD, reviews of the research on PMS in general and on PMDD or LLPDD specifically showed in great detail how deeply flawed most of it was. It is especially disturbing that the *DSM-IV* committee on LLPDD spent months putting together a lengthy review of research reports in which they concluded that the studies had been filled with methodological problems and that the existing research was in any case very preliminary, and yet the *DSM-IV* Task Force's recommendation was to keep LLPDD in the handbook and even to list it in the main text under "Depressive Disorders." This last move was all the more unscientific because even their own review did not yield much research that bore on the question of depression. So Judith Gold and her colleagues produced a research review that you would never in a million years expect to lead to a recommendation for keeping LLPDD in the handbook at all, never mind putting it under "Depression" in the main text. First of all, they reported that their review emphasized studies in which women kept daily symptom ratings for at least one menstrual cycle, but LLPDD is supposed to require two months' worth. Thus, most of the research they discuss does not even meet the criterion they chose for their review. Second, although their list of methodological problems in the literature runs almost two pages in length, they do not bring consideration of those to bear as they go on to evaluate each study. Third, all of the studies they reviewed in their "biological studies" section are about PMS, not LLPDD; thus, what sparse information there is, is about physical problems such as breast tenderness, not the mood changes that are supposed to be the key features of LLPDD. Furthermore, all but two of those studies were done before LLPDD was even proposed (and thus its criteria had not been selected), and even the two exceptions were poorly done. Each antidepressant mentioned in the review was tested in only a single study, and the numbers of people tested were very small. Finally, these four excerpts from their review make it crystal clear that LLPDD cannot be considered a legitimate construct:

> As is the case with most disorders in DSM-III-R, there are no explicit guidelines regarding how these clinical decisions are made. . . .
> The criteria as proposed in DSM-III-R do not offer sufficient guidelines for determining whether clinical worsening during the late luteal phase of the menstrual cycle reflects an exacerbation of another condition or superimposed LLPDD. . . .

The distinction between affective responsiveness and "emotional lability," a DSM-III-R criterion for the LLPDD disorder, cannot be made with validity or reliability. . . .

There are still only a small number of reports in the published literature using DSM-III-R criteria, including two months of prospective symptom ratings. . . . there is little evidence that even two months is sufficient to establish a menstrual-cycle-related disease.

In fact, there have been a few carefully done pieces of relevant research that shed some light on the subject. It has been shown, for example, that the more a woman believes in menstrual distress, the more she tends to exaggerate the negativity of her symptoms during her previous period when she is asked to recall them, and emotions reported retrospectively are described as more negative than emotions reported at the time they are experienced. Just knowing that one is participating in a study of the menstrual cycle can increase reports of negative symptoms by 80 percent. When women are asked to keep ratings *as they go* rather than to recall them, it turns out that physical symptoms, but few or no emotional ones, vary with cycle phase. Similarly, when women have been told that they are premenstrual, they report having more symptoms than when they have been told that they are intermenstrual. Indeed, even in women who have been diagnosed as "having LLPDD," cycle phase accounted for only 7 percent of mood changes, and for women who report that, as the *DSM* criteria specify, their premenstrual mood changes "seriously interfere" with their work or relationships, these reports are not borne out by more objective measures. In fact, women who report having premenstrual distress typically underestimate their performance on tasks and in some cases actually show more task persistence and more positive mothering behavior premenstrually than postmenstrually. When researchers compared mood stability in women who do and women who do not take contraceptive pills, as well as in men, no sex differences were found, although women not on the pills reported feeling more pleasant than did the other women or the men. Finally, women who have been given the LLPDD label tend to be characterized more by problems with self-esteem and ways of coping with stress and by sparse social supports than by premenstrual mood changes. All of these findings show how unwarranted is the claim that there is such a phenomenon as a premenstrual mental disorder.

As we thought about the research on SDPD and LLPDD, and especially as we contrasted it with the massive amounts of research supporting the DDPD category that the *DSM* people rejected, doctoral student Kaye Lee Pantony and I wondered whether the *DSM*'s aura of scientific precision was unjustified only in regard to gender-skewed categories or whether it was also bad for quite different categories. We decided to do some further investigating of our own, specifically looking at whether there was research to justify some of the other categories, the criteria for those categories, and their respective cutoff points. Put another way, this meant asking

- whether the research confirmed the existence of such mental disorders as those represented by the labels of the categories we chose to study;
- whether research had made it possible to discover the actual elements, or criteria, of each disorder; and

- whether research had made it possible to discover exactly how many criteria a person had to meet in order to belong clearly to a particular category.

Aiming for a wide variety of diagnoses, Pantony and I chose to examine three categories that could be applied to people of either sex. We selected two categories that are used for children—Autistic Disorder (AD) and Oppositional Defiant Disorder (ODD)—because SDPD and LLPDD are used for adults. We also chose Obsessive Compulsive Disorder (OCD), since it is used for both children and adults. (AD is an Axis II, Developmental Disorder; ODD is listed under "Other Disorders of Infancy, Childhood, or Adolescence," and it is not clear on which axis it belongs; and OCD is an Axis I disorder, although the more pervasive form, Obsessive Compulsive *Personality* Disorder, would go on Axis II.) Together with the work that my students and I had already done on SDPD and LLPDD, this would give us a total of five categories, with a substantial range of types of alleged mental disorders, whose scientific bases we would have examined.

Pantony scrupulously studied the research literature, using comprehensive computer searches to find studies that might be relevant. The searches covered approximately thirteen hundred periodicals and technical reports published throughout the world in more than twenty languages from mental health and related fields. The articles were published between 1967 and 1990, because we wanted to find out what empirical studies had been available when the decisions had been made to place these diagnostic categories in the *DSM*. Through a combination of computer searches and Pantony's diligence, we located a total of 351 articles relevant to the three categories.

In view of all of that research, we were frankly amazed

to find that *not a single empirically based article included any evidence of what the cutoff point for any of these categories ought to be.* In other words, there was no research on which to base the *DSM*'s prescriptions about how many criteria a person had to meet in order to be given any of those three labels: AD, ODD, or OCD. Those prescriptions cannot be said to have been derived from any scientific work whatsoever. In fact, the only article we located in which the selection of a cutoff point was even mentioned was in regard to the category of "Autism," and it was about the *lack of agreement* among clinicians about what cutoff point should be used in applying that label.

From the 220 articles we located that were about "Autistic Disorder," we found empirical support for including only two of the six criteria listed in the *DSM*. In other words, there is no empirical evidence that four of the six characteristics listed as features of autistic children are in fact features of autistic children. Of course, "Autism" is a construct, so there may not *be* any such phenomenon. Stated a bit differently, the research literature shows that there is no evidence that any more than two of the six *DSM* criteria for the category even tend to appear in the same person at the same time if at least one psychiatrist has diagnosed that child as autistic. In spite of this, in the *DSM* one finds a list of six criteria that are presented as frequent features of allegedly autistic children, and one also finds that such children have to have all six of the criteria in order to receive the label.

In the 124 articles we found that were related to Obsessive Compulsive Disorder, we found 92 that included some empirical research. However, in not a single article was there any attempt to document whether *any* of the *DSM*'s OCD criteria are actually important features of people with OCD (however one defines "OCD"), nor was there any empirical evidence bearing on the question of where the cutoff point should be.

We located only seven articles in which Oppositional Defiant Disorder was mentioned, and although most of them were based on empirical work, not one was addressed to the selection of criteria or of the cutoff point for ODD.

The various reviews of the SDPD and LLPDD literatures had also turned up no evidence that would have supported either the inclusion of any of the specific criteria in their respective lists or the choice of cutoff point for either category.

All told, then, there was little or no scientific evidence to justify the ways the criteria and cutoff points were chosen for a wide variety of *DSM* categories. It seems possible but highly unlikely that more rigorous standards were used for the categories that we happened not to study.

It is fascinating, though disturbing, to inspect the *DSM-IV* and observe the many instances of apparent, but unfounded, scientific precision. Under the category of "Encopresis," or lack of bowel control, the authors have constructed subtypes "based on whether or not constipation with overflow incontinence is present," but there is no evidence that there are meaningful psychological differences between people who are encopretic with and people who are encopretic without that added feature. In another show of scientific precision, "Selective Mutism" now requires a duration of one month. Is someone who has been mute for three weeks likely to be significantly different emotionally from someone who has been mute for thirty days? Similar time criteria are required for Brief Psychotic Disorder (now one day rather than the previous requirement of a few hours), Manic Episode (in *III*, a week's duration was required; in *III-R*, no duration was specified;

and in *IV*, it's back to a week). (Note here how different psychological categories are from true medical problems: A broken bone is a broken bone, pneumonia is pneumonia, whether one has had the break or the illness for three weeks or a month.)

In *IV*, Hypomanic Episode is contrasted to Manic Episode, which must last at least one week, the former lasting only at least four days and not being severe enough to cause significant impairment or to require hospitalization. What is one to do, then, about a problem of three days' duration that involves significant impairment?

With the *DSM-IV*, not only good science but even simple, logical thinking sometimes flies out the window. The category "Major Depressive Episodes with Atypical Features" includes "sensitivity to rejection"—hardly atypical for a depressed person. And a depressive episode is described as "Major" when, for instance, depression persists two months after the loss of a loved one. Instead, I should think, one might worry if depression has gone as soon as two months after a loved one's death. The six-month time limit allowed for adjustment to a major source of stress under "Adjustment Disorder" similarly means that massive numbers of people adjusting to unemployment, divorce, or immigration are pathologized for having difficulty lasting half a year. One does not want to believe that therapists can only understand people's reactions to situations if they have experienced such situations directly, but apparently that is sometimes the case. For such professionals, the *DSM*'s guidelines about when one crosses the line and becomes "disordered" do not help and can be hurtful to patients who are told their reactions are beyond the pale.

There are more examples of the lack of clarity in the *DSM* authors' thinking. They say that the diagnosis of Stereotypic Movement Disorder (in infants, children, or adolescents) should be given if the stereotypic movements or self-injuring behavior are severe enough to be focused on in treatment. According to this kind of reasoning, one does not determine if there is a problem and then treat it; instead, if one finds one is treating a kind of behavior, then it is a problem within the "mental disorder" category. And the authors seem to sense the primitive state of their field, because they felt it necessary to instruct users of the handbook that manic episodes that are clearly caused by antidepressant drugs should be diagnosed as "substance-induced manic episodes" rather than "Bipolar Disorder" (what used to be called "Manic-Depressive Disorder").

I am at a loss to explain a major change they made in the description of "Posttraumatic Stress Disorder," which I used to consider a potentially helpful diagnosis, because in *DSM-III-R* it included the remark that the disorder was caused by an experience (such as war or severe abuse) that would be traumatic for anyone. That remark accurately and helpfully normalized many people's experiences of panic, flashbacks, and difficulties in concentrating when they had been seriously traumatized. However, in the *DSM-IV*, the disorder is suddenly limited to problems caused by the person having experienced, witnessed, or been confronted with death or serious physical injury or a threat of such a consequence. In one fell swoop, the authors have denied the deeply traumatizing consequences of extreme verbal and emotional abuse. This move makes it far more likely that men (as war veterans) than women (severely emotionally abused by spouses or bosses) can make use of this diagnosis in seeking compensation for trauma. Furthermore, because this was the only category that had been described as an understandable and likely reaction to trauma, more women are now likely to be deprived of compassion and understanding. The clear implication of the change in this category is that psychological problems are understandable only as consequences of *physical* threats and harm.

I have belonged to groups in which political agendas and power dynamics influenced what went on but in which decisions were ultimately based on scientific research or careful logic. It may be impossible in any project to eliminate politics and power altogether, but groups do vary greatly in the values and standards they choose to guide their choices for action. As the evidence makes clear, the *DSM* players have chosen neither science nor logic—nor very much concern about the harm they do—as grounds for their choices.

The Gatekeeping Techniques

Combining our information about what the *DSM* group does (Chapters 4, 5, and 6) with our information about what it does *not* do (reported thus far in this chapter), psychologist June Larkin and I decided to write a descriptive summary of the "gatekeeping" techniques they use to control which categories go into the handbook and which stay out. We based this description solely on the material we had straight from the task force itself: its minutes, its formal publications, and letters its members had sent to me about SDPD, LLPDD, and DDPD. Although we cannot be sure that they use these gatekeeping techniques across the board, and although we may have failed to notice some gatekeeping methods in the materials we inspected, we aimed to make a start at identifying the techniques and exposing them to public scrutiny.

Even in our very limited materials, we found twenty-five different gatekeeping techniques that the *DSM* authors have used to keep concentrated in their hands the power to decide who is normal. (The complete list of twenty-five is presented in Table 1.) They included simply ignoring inquiries, such as questions about their deadlines and requests for copies of the unpublished studies they planned to consider in evaluating the controversial categories; ignoring information provided to them that supported categories they seemed to want excluded from the manual or that called into question categories they seemed to want included; disclosing only partial information (such as sending, at last, only some of the unpublished studies and not disclosing that there were more); breaking promises to send materials and information; using high or even impossibly high standards for research relating to diagnoses they appeared to dislike, while using laughably lax ones for those they favored; contradicting themselves and then failing to respond when asked to clarify the contradictions; using name-calling, especially calling those who disagreed with them "polemical" and "political," while flatly denying the highly political aspects of their own work; stacking the deck in their favor by ensuring that *DSM* honchos and supporters would have power to decide which articles about the manual would appear in major mental health publications, such as the *American Journal of Psychiatry* and less formal APA publications that are sent to the entire APA membership; lying outright, such as by denying that they said what they in fact had said in public; making patronizing psychological interpretations of their opponents' motives rather than responding to the merit of their concerns; and generally using a double standard for categories they appeared to like and those they appeared to dislike.

The double standard they have often used is to exclude diagnoses they consider undesirable by claiming that "new diagnoses should be included in the system only after they have proven themselves through research rather than being included to stimulate that research," even though they justify including or keeping such categories as LLPDD in the manual *on the grounds that they must be included to stimulate research.*

Another of their frequent gatekeeping techniques has been to contrast their allegedly rational, calm, scientific approach with the allegedly emotional, agitated, hurried, unscientific approach of their opponents. Responding to my paper "How *Do* They Decide Who Is Normal?" Frances and his colleagues wrote that they themselves were proceeding with "care and comprehensiveness," whereas I was trying to rush them into decisions before they had had a chance to weigh the evidence judiciously. They implied that those who disagreed with them had created "controversies that detract from the objective evaluation of the evidence and trivialize and personalize the process of developing the classification." They wrote further that they were engaged in "quiet consideration of the evidence" rather than what we were doing, which amounted to producing "a polemical expression of... personal views." This last statement is particularly interesting in light of the fact that what we had sent to them consisted almost entirely of detailed presentation and analysis of the relevant data, logical argumentation, and description of known dangers of their pet categories.

It is probably clear by now that the *DSM* group's gatekeeping techniques were driven not by a commitment to a logical, scientific approach and to the welfare of their patients but rather by a set of fairly obvious values. In their Personality Disorders Work Group's minutes from its September 1991 meeting, I noted that they had at last discussed—and rejected—DDPD and that they also discussed a proposal they had received for "Racist Personality Disorder." I have seen no references in any of their minutes to a new category that psychologist Arthur Nikelly had proposed to them, which he called "Pleonectic Personality Disorder," an obsession with material possessions. It is apparent that the *DSM* authors' gatekeeping techniques grow from a value system in which intense preoccupation with certain aspects of sexuality and with such practices as ritual handwashing are thought to deserve the label "mental disorder" but intense preoccupation with—and behavior persistently based on—racist, woman-hating, or deeply materialistic attitudes and beliefs are not. Is this a value system that we are comfortable using as the basis for defining who is and who is not normal?

With all of the false claims about the scientific integrity of the *DSM*, it is not surprising but it is worrying that the claims are passed on by others as though they were true. In *The New Harvard Guide to Psychiatry*, in a chapter called "Psychiatry and Society," Ming Tsuang, Mauricio Tohen, and Jane Murphy say, "*DSM-III-R*'s . . . highly specific operational criteria have made comparability in case identification an achievable goal." This is not true, of course, because the inter-rater reliability is so poor that the categories are of little value for comparative purposes.

I would like to give the penultimate word on the handbook's unwarranted aura of scientific precision to Matthew Dumont, a psychiatrist who has written about the *DSM* Work Group's hollow pretensions to scientific authority:

> I read the [DSM-III-R] compiler's Introduction (will I be the only person in the civilized world, except for a few copy editors, to have done so?) and found

it an interesting statement, part apologia, part three imperious knocks from the wings. The humility and the arrogance in the prose are almost indistinguishable, frolicking like puppies at play. They say: ". . . while this manual provides a classification of mental disorder . . . no definition adequately specifies precise boundaries for the concept . . ." [APA, 1987]. They then provide a 125-word definition of mental disorder which is supposed to resolve all the issues surrounding the sticky problem of where deviance ends and dysfunction begins. It doesn't.

They go on to say: ". . . there is no assumption that each mental disorder is a discrete entity with sharp boundaries between it and other mental disorders or between it and no mental disorder" [APA, 1987].

This is a remarkable statement in a volume whose 500-odd pages are devoted to the criteria for distinguishing one condition of psychopathology from another with a degree of precision indicated by a hundredth of a decimal place.

The final word—which strikes me as staggeringly ironic, although I am sure its author did not intend it that way—comes from John McIntyre, the APA's 1993–94 president, whose words begin the APA's advertising flyer and order form for the *DSM-IV*: "Perhaps no other work in APA history has been the subject of such rigorous review as has *DSM-IV*."

Table 1. *DSM-IV* Authors' Gatekeeping Techniques

1. Not responding to requests for
   (i) information regarding deadlines and procedures,
   (ii) copies of unpublished studies which only they had in their possession (or who they knew had them)

(iii) the bibliography they had put together and planned
to use for their literature review—although they
were sent a bibliography early on by Caplan and
Gans;

2. later, sending *some* of the unpublished studies but not
stating that those were not the only ones they intended
to use in their own review;

3. promising to send Caplan their own review of the SDPD
literature but delaying doing so until after *their* deadline
for receiving feedback on their review had passed;

4. claiming to have high standards for empirical research
to support their DSM decisions—but only applying those
standards to new diagnoses they don't want to include;

5. claiming that Caplan and Gans' review of the literature
(on SDPD) arrived too late to be considered in their
deliberations . . . ;

6. contradicting previous statements: For example, after
writing that Caplan and Gans' review had not been considered by the committee, Gunderson wrote in a later
letter that the review had been "an important source of
material for the discussion we had about the fate
of . . . SDPD" (Gunderson, letter to Caplan, October
16, 1989);

7. telling Caplan, within several days, both that SDPD
would probably stay in the *DSM-IV* and that it probably
would not;

8. dismissing the review by Caplan and Gans by calling it
polemical . . . ;

9. having some people who are in high positions on the
DSM Revisions Task Force also belong to the editorial
boards of journals where these issues ought to be aired;

10. not informing the feminist/critical reviewers about each
other's work (either while the reviews were being written
or after they were completed—thus failing to save these
reviewers time and effort, and thus making it more difficult for the reviewers to join forces with each other);

11. falsely attacking Caplan and Gans' critique (e.g., claiming
that Spitzer has never said the *DSM* categories are based
on good research, although Caplan and Gans had cited
the place in the *DSM* version edited by Spitzer where he
said they were);

12. making psychological interpretations of Caplan's objections instead of treating them on their merits ...;

13. asserting divine or natural right for the *DSM* process: "I think we should let nature take its course" ...;

14. saying there is little enthusiasm [in the Work Group on Personality Disorders] for SDPD while actually preparing detailed modifications of the specific criteria and justifications for them;

15. questioning the seriousness of Caplan and Eichler's intentions in proposing DDPD as a diagnostic category;

16. saying they would review the empirical work (on DDPD) if Caplan and Eichler would assemble it, although their own people do the literature reviews for other categories;

17. refusing to specify the exact standards and criteria which they use in deciding whether to include or exclude categories;

18. dismissing with no explanation Caplan's point that there is a great deal of existing research which is relevant to DDPD;

19. explicitly discouraging the DDPD authors by following up a comment about the need for Caplan and Eichler to provide empirical support for DDPD with the statement that "if this sounds discouraging, I'm afraid it is meant to" (Frances, letter to Caplan, July 24, 1989, p. 1);

20. insinuating that the DDPD authors would not *want* to provide them with the empirical support for DDPD, although they had offered to do so;

21. dismissing DDPD before seeing the relevant review of the literature;

22. failing to assign any Task Force member to coordinate the review of the DDPD category;

23. stating that they are against adding new diagnostic categories;

24. claiming to be unaware of research relevant to DDPD, although the DDPD authors had informed members of the *DSM-IV* Revisions Task Force about that research and mentioned those bodies of literature in a letter to them;

25. dismissing the research on violence against women, attri-

bution theory, and many other topics as irrelevant to DDPD while continuing to include research on "masochism" as "support" for SDPD despite the differences in criteria for masochism and SDPD.

8

What Motivates the *DSM* Authors?

People frequently ask me, "Why do the *DSM* authors make their decisions as they do? Why don't they listen to reason, take research into account, and worry about the effects their decisions have on patients?" During the first years after I became acquainted with some of the *DSM* authors, I believed that they genuinely felt that their choices were most likely to help their patients. I thought, of course, that they were wrong about that, but I wanted to regard their motives as honorable. In the past few years, although I continue to think that some of them really do believe they are making responsible decisions, I have reluctantly come to recognize that some of their motives are probably far less honorable.

When Robert Spitzer earnestly told a women's magazine reporter during the press conference at the 1986 APA convention that psychiatrists needed to have LLPDD in the handbook so that they could do research and find out how best to help women, I assumed he was being sincere. My lifelong wish to regard those in authority as well-meaning and intelligent made it easier for me to cling to that assumption. Neither then nor even now have I known any of the major players very well, and I certainly have never known any of them outside the context of discussions and debates about psychiatric diagnosis, so everything I am about to say is conjecture. It's hard enough to understand fully what one's own motives are for taking any action or holding a particular belief, and it is virtually impossible to know for certain what motivates anyone else. The following, then, are speculations; when I have some reason other than my own ideas for naming a particular source of motivation for one or more of the *DSM* authors, I present that reason.

My main conclusion: The sheer mass of evidence that the major players in the *DSM* continually ignore both the research and the harm suffered by patients due to the handbook's categories is incompatible with their being driven by only the most altruistic and balanced of motives. Something is very wrong when those at the top of the *DSM* hierarchy not only ignore scientific evidence and ignore proof of the harm they are doing but also admit (see Chapter 4) that they don't want their patients to know what goes on in *DSM* meetings. That they would spontaneously make such remarks to those of us who were energetically opposing their moves suggests either a whopping case of arrogance and sense of privilege or an astonishing naivete—and the latter seems highly unlikely. In my book *You're Smarter Than They Make You Feel: How the Experts Intimidate Us and What We Can Do about It*, I considered the question of why all kinds of experts and authorities neglect or mistreat the people they are supposed to serve, and many of the possible answers to that question apply to the *DSM* people. I shall start with the kinds of motives that would encourage us to give them the benefit of the doubt, and then I shall move toward the less complimentary ones.

As I have said, from my own experience as a twenty-two-year-old trainee in a clinical psychology doctoral program, I know that it can feel quite overwhelming suddenly to be expected to function as a therapist and, therefore, to know how to help people who are suffering. It is even more disconcerting to feel, as many therapy supervisors and even many patients make us feel, that we are supposed to know and understand more about the patients than they know and understand about themselves. Under these circumstances, it is not surprising that people in training programs for social work, psychology, psychiatric nursing, counseling, and psychiatry often cope with these feelings by turning to their teachers and to the writings of acknowledged experts to see how they should act and what they should believe about how to deal with their patients. They become trapped within the theories and procedures that they have been taught, unable to break out of those frameworks. Most people find it difficult to tolerate uncertainty and want to believe that their work is helpful and effective. The most caring decision makers need to believe that what they are doing is right because they know that many people who seek therapy are suffering greatly, and sometimes the sources of their suffering are hard to pinpoint or seem impossible to change; so to be able to resort to textbook-style instructions about how to categorize and treat can be reassuring. At best, then, some of the people who put together the handbook may genuinely be trying to help but are unquestioningly following teachings that are not helpful or are frankly harmful to patients, under the misguided notion that what they are doing is the best that can be done for their patients. It is disconcerting to recognize that one may not really be helping one's patients, and examining what one does might bring one face to face with that sad fact.

Another motive that may impel some or all of the *DSM* authors is that, if they have never been therapy patients themselves (in most training programs, therapists are not required to undergo therapy) or have never had the most damaging diagnostic labels applied to them, they may simply not stop to think carefully about the effects their decisions will have on millions of patients. This could grow out of mental laziness, fear of being in patients' shoes, or both. In regard to the latter, it can feel dangerous to think too vividly about patients' experiences, because one might discover that even patients branded with labels that make them seem bizarre are not all that different from oneself.

A less admirable aim that might be motivating some of the *DSM* authors is the wish to appear professional and knowledgeable by being in step with those of their predecessors and contemporary colleagues who have become famous and influential. To be an agent of enshrining the pronouncements of the latter in the official diagnostic handbook can be to gain respectability for oneself. Some members of the handbook task force may want not only this increased respectability per se but also the rewards that accompany support for those in power. These can include referrals of patients, job offers, requests to write for or edit prestigious professional journals, increased income, and fame.

Quite apart from the power, wealth, and fame that can come from allegiance to those who are already influential through their writings and teachings, simply being a member of the *DSM* hierarchy can provide power and control. Your name appears in numerous widely read professional publications and, if you are close enough to the top, quite likely will appear in the mass media. This tends to bring large numbers of calls from people who want you to be their therapist. Indeed, the February 1994 issue of *Good*

Housekeeping magazine contains a list that is purported to be composed of the names of the best therapists in their fields; it includes a large proportion of those who have been most prominent in *DSM* decision-making procedures.

Some people may be motivated by the enjoyment of having so much power to make decisions about who is not normal. Furthermore, as their actual practice has shown, the top players in the *DSM* game have the enormous power to overlook the evidence of scientific research and the documentation of harm done by their work, and they have the power to choose not to use logical or humane principles in making their decisions. For some people, these kinds of power, this freedom from rules and standards, are intoxicating.

I list the desire to make money as a motive at this point not because I believe it is less admirable than the drive for power and control (they can all lead to devastating consequences for the people they are supposed to serve) but because it is one of the least admirable and because there is a great deal of evidence that it plays an important role in the operation of the *DSM* Task Force and the workings of the American Psychiatric Association overall. To begin with, the *DSM* is a huge moneymaker. The previous edition brought in one million dollars, and every time a new edition appears, libraries, therapists, general practitioners, and researchers have to throw out the old ones and purchase the new. Furthermore, the more diagnostic categories there are, the more potential patients there are and, therefore, the more income there is for psychiatrists. Sometimes, official APA doctrine includes unabashed statements to that effect, as when the unnamed author(s) of the March 1994 *DSM-IV Update* wrote that a new category called Bipolar II Disorder, like some others, had been added to the manual "because it increases diagnostic coverage." I find it so personally distasteful to think of financial motives as driving work that is advertised as intended to help alleviate people's suffering that this was the last motive I found myself able to attribute to anyone connected with the handbook and the APA. However, it is undeniable that the increase from fewer than 300 to 374 "mental disorders" between *III-R* and *IV* allows therapists who so wish to sweep far more patients—with their fees—into their treatment circle. Furthermore, mental health researchers have money to gain, because of "the tendency for research funding to follow the establishment of diagnostic categories."

What began to make me particularly suspicious was the pattern of the *DSM* advocates' defense of LLPDD in the 1993 protest. The *only* kind of "treatment" they proposed to the public—and they mentioned it every time they had the chance—was the use of antidepressant medications. Occasionally, Judith Gold would admit, if asked, that changes in diet and nutrition, as well as exercise and self-help groups (hardly the stuff of psychiatric disorders), had been shown to help women who felt they had mood problems premenstrually, but it was clear that the only *psychiatric* treatment they could offer was to give the women psychotropic drugs. It turns out, of course, that a huge proportion of the research on LLPDD that Robert Spitzer claimed was so urgently needed in order to learn how to help women has been and will likely be funded by the drug companies that have everything to gain, in both money and respectability, from the *DSM* Task Force's decision about LLPDD. Psychologist Mary Brown Parlee has said, for instance, that drug companies have pushed for the treatment of "PMS" as a medical problem. She has noted that pharmaceutical houses "stand to make a great deal of money if every menstruating woman could take a few pills every month. Drug companies sponsor research conferences and 'medical education' seminars on PMS," events, she says, "for which they actively and effectively seek media coverage." "It is to the drug companies' interest," she adds, "if physicians and the public confuse the small minority of women who have premenstrual or menstrual problems with the majority who have normal, undrugworthy menstrual cycles." And psychologist Carol Tavris observes similarly that menopause is "too big a market to remain undiagnosed and untreated." Those *DSM* Task Force members who hope to receive drug company funding for their own research or who aim to attract more such monies to psychiatric research in general will have a stake in increasing the number of categories in the manual, since each category is supposed to be "researchable." At a recent meeting about the *DSM*, a consultant for the handbook reported that a drug company is currently showing intense interest in funding a planned Canadian study, speculating that the topic of the research will appear in the *DSM-IV-R*, *V*, or whatever the next edition will be called. Once a category appears in the manual, of course, it becomes much easier to sell therapists and patients on the notion that drug treatment is appropriate.

My suspicion was increased when I read a statement in the *Archives of General Psychiatry* by Dr. Mark Zimmerman, a psychiatrist who assisted with *DSM-III-R* revisions:

> Appendix D in *DSM-III-R* lists the reasons for the changes [from *DSM-III* to *DSM-III-R*], and it is noteworthy that only a minority were based on accumulated research. Having sat on the melancholia subcommittee and kept closely informed of the

changes in the personality disorder section, I saw firsthand the oftimes unscientific nature by which changes were made in the official diagnostic criteria . . . the changes in the criteria were not data-based. . . . If science can have only a minimal impact on the revision of *DSM-III-R*, then what else might be driving the system? More specifically, to what extent are financial considerations beneficial to the APA—and hence all of us—perhaps responsible for the urgency to publish yet another edition? I have asked these questions of some of the *DSM-IV* task [force] members and they too have heard such concerns, and they *hoped* that financial motives were not primarily responsible for the urgency. I hope so too.

Indeed, it turns out that "The drug companies provide the backbone of financial support for APA." Psychiatrist Peter Breggin has written extensively about this subject and reports:

The psychiatric newspapers and journals, including those published by APA, are largely paid for by drug company advertising. In 1987, for example, the APA newspaper *Psychiatric News* had a surplus of $1,311,554, largely the result of drug ads. In recent years, according to its annual reports published each October in the *American Journal of Psychiatry*, 15 to 20 percent of APA's total revenue has come from drug company advertising.

Breggin goes on to report that drug companies give several million dollars each year to underwrite APA's national conferences and indeed that APA probably could not afford to put on those conferences without that money. The drug companies also support such political projects as

APA's annual meetings about lobbying for legislation that is favorable to psychiatrists. When questioned by Breggin about the APA–drug company connection, an APA bigwig—Daniel Freedman, who had edited the *Archives of General Psychiatry* for twenty years—called concerns about the connection "Marxist" and "paranoid."

Psychiatrists other than Breggin have spoken out about these concerns. A top APA official, Fred Gottlieb, wrote a report for the APA's *American Journal of Psychiatry* in which he expressed his concern about research demonstrating that physicians' prescribing of drugs is powerfully affected by "commercial sources" such as drug companies. Gottlieb called a section of his report "Better Living Through Chemistry: Industry Money for Education and Amenities" and pointed out that the APA's own Scientific Program Committee had written to the APA president to express concern about the effects the drug companies were having on allegedly scientific programming.

In his candidacy statement when he ran for APA president, Dr. Paul Fink apparently assumed his words would be well received when he said baldly, "It is the task of APA to protect the earning power of psychiatrists." As Breggin summarizes the point:

> organized psychiatry is big business more than it is a profession. As a big business, managed by APA and NIMH, it develops media relationships, hires PR firms, develops its medical image, holds press conferences to publicize its products, lobbies on behalf of its interests, and issues "scientific" reports that protect its members from malpractice suits by lending legitimacy to brain-damaging technologies. It tries to increase not only its share of the market, but also the size of the whole market.

Insurance companies feed psychiatrists' concern with diagnosis as a route to financial gain when they pay for treatment only if a patient receives a formal diagnosis (perhaps even only one from the *DSM*) or only certain diagnoses from within a classification system. As a result, therapists may find themselves using a diagnostic system, or particular diagnostic labels, so that they will be paid for their services as much as because the system makes sense or the labels are appropriate. This would not be problematic if the only result were that people needing help got that help. But, as noted, with labeling always goes the gamut of dangers, from the patient feeling shame about supposedly being mentally ill to problems in obtaining employment to losing a range of legal rights.

On the general subject of the wish of some psychiatrists to stay on top of the heap, whether that is important to them for reasons of money, reasons of power and status, or both, psychiatry as a profession is clearly concerned about having to compete for patients with all of the other kinds of therapists. So, say Kirk and Kutchins, where psychiatrists had "won cultural jurisdiction over personal problems from the clergy and from neurologists by the middle of this century," they now "constitute less than 20% of all mental health professionals." Joseph English, then APA president, reported in 1993, "Our goal has been to develop a strategic plan that would help APA . . . achieve parity with other medical disorders" and described their "strategic plan" to "improve the public image of psychiatry," noting, "Most importantly, I am delighted to report to you that Ann Landers, after a period of disillusionment, is once again recommending psychiatrists, when they are needed, to her 90 million readers. I can think of no better indicator of progress related to our efforts in public affairs." The more psychiatrists keep the public believing that only medically trained personnel can deal fully with people's personal problems, the greater chance they will have of attracting the lion's share of the potential patient population. The *DSM* serves this purpose well.

Kirk and Kutchins also believe that psychiatry as a profession needs to shore up the precariousness of its position because it sits "at the bottom of the totem pole of medical specialties," partly because mental health professionals from nonmedical disciplines do so much of the same work as psychiatrists. Producing the diagnostic handbook, say sociologists Phil Brown and Elizabeth Cooksey, enables psychiatry to dominate other mental health professions and to "solidif[y] the claim that it is 'hard' medicine worthy of government support for education and services, and for third party reimbursement." This latter aim is increasingly important amidst debates about what health insurance should cover.

What persuades me of the power-hungry nature of many of those who hold the most powerful positions within all of the mental health professions is their unresponsiveness to requests and recommendations from groups of consumers of mental health services and of other groups, such as women's groups. I was a co-author of the Canadian Mental Health Association's report *Women and Mental Health in Canada*, in which we made a large number of highly specific recommendations for improving women's mental health. Many of these recommendations were directed at training programs for all kinds of psychotherapists, but they have been almost totally ignored by directors of almost all such programs.

The motives discussed so far could apply to anyone involved in the general project of producing diagnostic categories, but when it comes to specific categories that are especially harmful to particular groups of people, different motives may be at work. For instance, those impelled by the wish to ignore the many social causes of women's unhappiness would find it useful to invoke Self-Defeating Personality Disorder to imply that individual women's unconscious needs lead them to bring misery on themselves. Those same diagnostic specialists would find Premenstrual Dysphoric Disorder a convenient way to attribute women's unhappiness to their hormones or some mysterious tie to a cycle of moods. Both categories make it easier to ignore such factors as the high rates of violence against girls and women, dramatic pay inequities, and unreasonable blame our socialization places on mothers as possible causes of women's sadness. From an historical perspective, it is pretty easy to predict when "PMS" comes in and out of public and professional attention. Carol Tavris has described in detail the way that "the idea that menstruation is a debilitating condition that makes women unfit for work . . . comes and goes in phase with women's participation in the labor market." The more that men need jobs, the stronger grows the emphasis on women's unfitness for the workforce due to alleged menstrual-related problems.

Another example of the use of *DSM* by those who wish to veil social problems relates to sexual abuse. Louise Armstrong has written that to focus on saying that male or female victims of severe abuse have "Borderline Personality Disorders" or "Multiple Personality Disorders" both swings the focus away from the perpetrator and treats the victims' psychological survival mechanisms as abnormal. Including "Ego Dystonic Homosexuality" in the manual after publicly announcing that it no longer considered homosexuality a mental illness could only have been done by people who believed either that our society does *not* make it difficult to live happily as a homosexual or that that difficulty does not matter. Indeed, the *DSM* as a whole discourages practitioners (or at least does little or nothing to encourage them) from exploring the social or political environments that cause people pain. Ignoring these admittedly complex forces, especially severe forms of bias and mistreatment, no doubt affords some therapists the inner peace that comes from believing that nothing that is happening within their purview requires them to speak up, to protest, to take social action, to take a risk.

I have been asked how the all-woman LLPDD committee could possibly have acted as it did. Again, I can only speculate. To begin with, we should remember that those who are chosen to serve as full members of *DSM* committees are usually—though not quite always—those who already share the views of the *DSM* leaders or those who long for power within APA. Then, it is important to remember that the LLPDD committee and its leader, Judith Gold, initially had the integrity *not* to pretend that they had reached a consensus about what to recommend. Once Andreasen and Rush had been called in and the *DSM* Task Force's official position became to include the category in both the appendix and the main text, Gold and some members of her committee publicly gave the impression that they—or the committee—fully supported that position (see Chapters 4 and 9). One member, Sally Severino, had the courage to continue expressing her reservations even after the official decision was publicized. It is not surprising, though it is disappointing, that some women will give personal power or the image of group unanimity a higher priority than honesty and concern about harm done to women as a result of their decisions.

The range of motives that might impel the *DSM* authors is considerable, but no matter what motive or mixture of motives might characterize each one of them, there is surely no excuse for their scientific irresponsibility and frequent ignoring of evidence of the harm that they do.

9

Media: The Good and the Bad

If the media had told the *DSM* story fairly and truthfully, I do not think it would have occurred to me to write this book. But after watching the *DSM* authors twist and hide the truth, then to watch so many media people continue that process was just too much. Because of my time as a reporter for a medium-sized Midwestern newspaper, as well as my natural inclinations, I suppose, I regarded the media as immensely valuable vehicles for public education. And in the twenty or so years that I have been giving interviews to media people, I had had very few disappointing experiences. All this changed, however, when I saw the media coverage of the *DSM* story.

To my knowledge, not a single U.S. evening news show and only one Canadian evening news show covered the story, and that surely would have been vastly different had the story been about pathologizing half a million men. During the 1992–93 protest against LLPDD/PMDD, I did more than fifty interviews and media appearances on the subject, including print media and radio and television shows. I have tried to obtain copies of all of the stories in which I was involved, and although I did not get all of them, I do have twenty-five newspaper (including newspaper columns as well as feature and news stories) and magazine articles (fifteen U.S., eight English-Canadian, one French-Canadian, and one British), described in Appendix A. I also have audiotapes of two U.S. and two Canadian radio programs, and videotapes of two U.S. and two Canadian television shows, listed in Appendix B. The main reason I want to focus on media coverage for which I was interviewed is that I know what I told the reporters and producers, so I can tell what they ignored or distorted.

From time to time, people speculate about whether, as a feminist, I am unduly suspicious of societal institutions and their seemingly inherent male biases. But the fact is that the print media reporters were overwhelmingly female—twenty-three women, three men (some articles were coauthored, so the number of writers is greater than the number of articles)—and of the eight broadcast journalists, seven were women and one was a man. I did find I was more surprised and disappointed when women failed to understand the issues than when men did, because women have so much more to lose. But as to the question of my being unduly suspicious, with regard to the media as with regard to the *DSM* players, I began by assuming that they were acting in good faith. I continue to believe that many of the reporters were not consciously distorting what I said. However, I have come to understand another significant factor, which is that the reporters and interviewers grew up in the same culture that produced the *DSM* authors, and so they, too, filter what they hear through their belief system. And one of the fundamental notions within the belief system in which we have all been immersed is that women are inferior, and that this is probably somehow linked to our essential femaleness and, therefore, to our "female" hormones. This filtering process makes it hard for them to understand how the evidence blatantly contradicts what the *DSM* people say, because the *DSM* view fits with the reporters' existing beliefs. For this reason, evidence contradicting previously accepted beliefs is difficult to believe and to write about. In a sense, I think it simply doesn't occur to them that there *could* be evidence that contradicts what the psychiatrists claim, since they assume that the psychiatrists' words are true. It is well known that it is harder to remember information that does not fit with one's beliefs than to remember information that supports them. Furthermore, as I have written elsewhere, most North Americans are raised to believe what so-called experts tell them and to doubt their own ability to ask intelligent questions and to challenge what the experts say. Although it is true that the essence of any reporter's work is supposed to be the asking of good, hard, probing questions and then following them up with more good questions, many reporters are like most other people with respect to the awe with which they regard authorities in fields that have languages laden with jargon, like the mental health field and especially research on mental health. Furthermore, I am continually struck by the reluctance of many people, including reporters, to ask challenging questions of those in the so-called helping professions, because they feel somehow that it is rude to question the motives of those who are described as dedicating their lives to serving others. Since we live in a generally sexist society, when the APA says it has decided to stop disbelieving women who say they have PMS and will now believe them—as long as they pay the price of being called mentally ill—it is hard for us to put our fingers on why that move is sexist. It seems, at first glance, that the APA is doing women a favor by now believing what women tell them.

Lack of awareness of the ways one's biases impede one's ability to think and write is hard to justify in reporters, but writing slanted stories without disclosing one's conflicts of interest is inexcusable. One writer who presented the *DSM* authors as scrupulously scientific apparently served in the Peace Corps with the man who was APA president at the time the former wrote his piece.

Although I hope it is now clear that I think the willfully distorting reporter is rare, I also think it is important to tell the most egregious instance of intentional manipulation of the story by media people for blatantly political, sexist purposes. In that story, the woman who interviewed me—and later told me about her bosses' manipulation of the reporting—warned me that she could lose her job if she were ever associated with this story, so I want it known that her coverage of the LLPDD events may or may not be listed in Appendix A, the list of print interviews, or Appendix B, the list of broadcast ones.

The reporter in question contacted me when she read in a newspaper article that I was trying to prevent the APA from keeping LLPDD in their handbook. She said that she wanted to do an extensive piece and would like to interview *DSM* task force members, some of the people working with me, and me. She also remarked at the outset that her personal belief was that the category had no place in a psychiatric manual. She interviewed a number of people on our side, including me, and also interviewed Judith Gold and others who shared Gold's attitudes. When the piece appeared, I told her that I was impressed by the sheer number of issues she had packed into it but was disappointed that she had included claims made by *DSM* people that she knew to be totally unfounded (such as that their recommendations were based on the research). I said I was especially surprised by this because I had given her so much concrete documentation to show clearly and simply that their claims were unjustified. I wondered, I said, whether she had been trying so hard to conceal her own opinion that she had gone to the other extreme.

The reporter sighed, was silent for a bit, and then told me the following story. When she had first proposed doing the piece, her bosses had flatly turned down her proposal. They were adamant about not letting her do anything about the issue. Some weeks later, U.S. and Canadian media prominently featured stories about politician Kim Campbell, who, it suddenly appeared, was highly likely to become Canada's first woman prime minister. At that point, the reporter's bosses called her in, expressed their alarm about the prospect of a woman holding such high political office, and told her to do the story, because "Maybe we can prove that Kim Campbell goes crazy once a month and shouldn't be Prime Minister of Canada!" She said that she had been lucky to sneak in the few arguments from our side that appeared in the final story.

In the pieces they produced, the vast majority of the reporters (with a very few striking exceptions) unquestioningly accepted the claims about normality that were made by *DSM* spokespeople. In each interview I provided documentation—in the forms of printed reports from the APA itself and of tapes of radio and television debates between APA personnel and myself—that no one has ever been able to produce *any* research to support the claim that PMS is a mental illness. I also provided evidence of the serious emotional, physical, social, and economic harm that women have suffered due to the classification of PMS as a psychiatric disorder (as described in Chapter 5). In spite of this, nearly every media story presented, as though it were truth, the notion that there is definitely a form of PMS that is a mental illness and gave the impression that research supported that view. Furthermore, although I provided indisputable documentation of the poor scientific methodology and the decision-making process about PMS that was filled with political games, apparent decisions to ignore the data, and cover-ups of the truth, most reporters concealed these facts. In effect, they treated statements from the APA as though they were the APA's press agents rather than performing the function of questioning or even of balanced reporting that the media are supposed to carry out.

In the name of "presenting both sides," media people commit many sins. That is because "presenting both sides" ought not to mean simply telling what Gold claimed and telling what Caplan claimed, if one has indisputable evidence that what Gold says is untrue. But, much though I hate to admit it, reporters may be no more intelligent or interested in thinking deeply and thoroughly than anyone else. And so, I believe, many persuade themselves that they are covering both sides when actually they are helping to promulgate the lies of one side by reporting them as though they were well-founded truths and failing to report the documentation that shows they are wrong.

The manifestations of bias in the media that I noticed in the case of the 1993 PMDD campaign were not unusual. Jean Hamilton, one of the early opponents of LLPDD/PMDD, was at the Institute for Research on Women's Health when she wrote about some of the same results of bias that she had observed in regard to media coverage of *DSM*-related issues. Parallel with the way reporters in the 1993 coverage often made our side appear politically motivated and unconcerned with science and the other side appear as though its motives and concerns were the opposite, she wrote that the attribution of "tainted motives operates as a powerful tool

for discounting women in science." She pointed out that
"a variety of women in science . . . made scientific, em-
pirically-based arguments in opposition to the PMS-re-
lated diagnosis (e.g., data on the inflation rate in self
reports, lack of needed controls, lack of cutoff criteria)"
and that "In contrast, many—if not most—of the arguments in support of the proposed diagnosis were non-
scientific (e.g., that the diagnosis would 'help' women;
that only a small number of women would be labelled;
that 'women' wanted the diagnosis, and so on)." Hamilton wrote,

> Nonetheless, an exact reversal of the actual posi-
> tions was portrayed prominently in both pro-
> fessional and mainstream media reports on the
> debate. That is, the opposition was mistakenly
> characterized as originating in *anonymous* and *non-
> scientific* "feminist groups" [Rovner, 1986]; in
> "*feelings* voiced by feminist groups" [Fink, 1987];
> and in "feminists" [dePaul, 1986] who exerted
> "feminist political pressures" [*The Psychiatric Times*,
> 1986].

Hamilton also noted the use of differently loaded terms
to describe *DSM* supporters and opponents:

> Instead of using a neutral term such as the "opposi-
> tion," scientists who opposed the diagnosis were
> labeled "antagonists" . . . ; and, instead of acknowl-
> edging a variety of scientifically based arguments,
> the antagonists were said simply to "complain," . . .
> causing otherwise "reasonable people . . . to turn
> their back on hard scientific evidence."

After I had been interviewed during those months in 1993, by reading through the articles and listening to and watching the tapes of stories about PMDD, I identified some of the good and some of the bad things the reporters (and, in some cases no doubt, their editors or producers) had done. I use "good" here to mean either that they made sure to include the documented facts I had given them or that they showed evidence of having thought logically and critically and followed through until they could make sense of contradictory arguments. I use "bad" to mean a failure to think logically and to ask either the other side or ours for support or proof to back up any claims that they/we might have made. A really good journalist would listen carefully to people on both sides for inconsistencies, unproven assertions, and contradictions and would doggedly ask questions in an attempt to find some resolution or at least some clarity. I find both irresponsible and distasteful the common practice of mindlessly transmitting the words of each side and leaving it to the reader to do the logical thinking. This is particularly disturbing because the reader usually cannot easily get in touch with the parties who were interviewed and do the questioning that the reporter should have done.

I analyzed the information from the print media separately from the information from the broadcast media. First I shall describe what I found in the published articles, and then I shall describe what happened on the radio and television programs. I classified the good and the bad practices of the print media people with whom I had contact and whose resulting pieces I could carefully review, and these are listed in Table 1. In the left column are the descriptions of those practices, and in the right column are the stories in which those practices were used. I listed as good practices anything I knew, from what I had told a reporter, to be an accurate portrayal. I listed as bad practices a reporter's failure to question a claim made by supporters of PMDD *only* when I had given the reporter concrete documentation to show that the supporters' claim was unfounded or dead wrong.

Table 1—Good and Bad Practices of Print Reporters

Good Practices	Print Article*
Makes it clear that a premenstrually related mental illness has not been proven to exist	2, 3, 6, 7, 9, 10, 11, 12, 13, 14, 20, 22
Makes it clear that feeling bad or upset is not the same thing as having a psychiatric disorder	2, 3, 11, 13, 14, 16, 18, 22
Describes harm that can result from use of the PMDD category	2, 3, 6, 7, 8, 10, 12, 14, 15, 16, 18, 19, 20, 22, 25
Reports the magnitude of the protest against the category	6
Reports that opponents of the category are protesting in part on scientific grounds	2, 3, 7, 20
Reports the lack of consensus about PMDD within the APA and even within the PMDD Work Group	7, 10, 11, 14, 17, 22, 24
Describes the nature and details of the dissension within the PMDD Work Group	7, 15
Describes how influential the *DSM* is outside the psychiatric community, and therefore the massive impact of its categories, despite APA personnel's denial of this	2, 8, 20
Describes the failure to find a biological basis for PMDD	2, 8, 18

*See Appendix A for listing of articles and the numbers that represent the respective articles in Table 1.

Good Practices *continued*	Print Article*
Describes the way that so-called PMS and PMDD mood symptoms are caused by socialization and situational factors	2, 3, 8, 9, 11, 22
Describes the double standard of pathologizing only women's hormonally based mood changes	2, 3, 9, 11, 14, 18, 22, 24, 25
Points out the absurdity of requiring only one mood or emotional symptom (and four common physical ones) in order to apply a psychiatric label	10, 23, 24
Presents evidence that a large number of women will receive this label	2, 10, 12
Reports that there is no concrete evidence that this label has helped women	10
Points out that it is strange to list the category title in the main text but the criteria only in the provisional appendix	21
Reports the heavily male percentages of members of the APA bodies that make *DSM* decisions	3, 20, 21
Points out the subjectivity involved in deciding whose lives are "markedly" interfered with by mood changes	2, 3, 20
Reports the sloppy *DSM* process and the confusion that often characterizes it	2, 20, 21, 22, 24
Reports the lack of scientific basis for listing PMDD in the main text specifically under Depression	2, 22

*See Appendix A for listing of articles and the numbers that represent the respective articles in Table 1.

Bad Practices	Print Article*
Fails to question the claim that good scientific evidence supports the existence of this category	4, 6, 17, 19, 20, 22, 23, 24
Reifies PMDD, writing about it as though it had been proven to exist and to be a mental disorder	11, 18, 20, 21, 23, 25
Fails to question the implication that there are only two options: for doctors and indeed everyone to ignore women's complaints of feeling bad or to call them mentally ill	4, 14, 15, 17, 24
Fails to question the claim that a woman must receive *this* diagnosis (rather than, say, the ordinary one of Depression) in order to be reimbursed by her insurance company for therapy	4, 23
Fails to report the scientific support and logical analysis behind claims of PMDD's opponents	4, 17
Fails to challenge PMDD supporters' false claims that the category is now, or has ever been, listed only in the provisional appendix	6, 11, 17, 23, 25
Uses loaded words to refer to opponents of the PMDD category	4, 15, 17, 22, 24
Ignores the real issues in the debate, treating it instead as though it were a catfight among women	5
Fails to ask for explanations or justifications of PMDD supporters' claims about its opponents	6
Fails to question supporters' claim that there is no evidence of women having been harmed by the label	6, 8, 11, 15, 17, 18, 20, 25
Quotes my remark that 14–45	6

*See Appendix A for listing of articles and the numbers that represent the respective articles in Table 1.

Bad Practices *continued*	Print Article*
percent of women complaining of PMS had gotten the PMDD diagnosis but fails to say that those figures came straight from the *DSM* work group's own research and publication	
Fails to question the claim that if PMDD is not in the manual, one cannot do research about it	7, 14, 17, 19, 22, 23
Fails to question supporters' claim that only a "tiny" group of women will be given the diagnosis	8, 11, 12, 15, 17, 23, 25
Fails to grasp and convey the point that for the label to appear in the main text is dangerous, even if the criteria are not listed there, and is bizarre	8, 20
Fails to grasp and convey the point that the huge amount of research that has been done has *still* failed to prove that there is a premenstrual mental illness and that, therefore, it would seem to be time to turf the category out of the handbook	8, 11, 19
Denies or fails to note the gender bias or double standard embodied in this category	8, 14, 18, 24
Conveys the outright lie from PMDD supporters that the research literature was conclusive	11
Fails to question or challenge supporters' attempt to respond to concerns about stigmatizing women by simply asserting that people ought not to stigmatize the mentally ill	11

*See Appendix A for listing of articles and the numbers that represent the respective articles in Table 1.

Bad Practices	Print Article*
Fails to question supporters' claim that 90 percent of women have PMS	11
Fails to question the claim that women "deserve" to get psychiatric treatment for "PMDD" and that such treatment works	11, 23
Fails to question supporters' claim that there was no dissension among them	17
Fails to question the claim that the diagnosis is needed in order to help women	17
Ignores the fact that a woman need have only one mood symptom to get the psychiatric diagnosis, while the rest can be everyday kinds of physical symptoms	17, 18, 20, 22, 24
Ignores the substantial role that subjectivity plays as therapists decide if a woman's moods "markedly interfere" in her life	17, 19, 20, 22, 25
Fails to question why, since hormone treatments don't help, the label would include the word "premenstrual"	18
Ignores the damning evidence that there is no such legitimate construct	20
Ignores the sloppy *DSM* process	20
Fails to question a supporter's complete lack of logic	24, 25

*See Appendix A for listing of articles and the numbers that represent the respective articles in Table 1.

The following examples will give a flavor of the kinds of poor reporting to which these various practices led.

Examples of Bad Reporting

In a *U.S. News and World Report* article, the writer, Erica Goode, could have been the *DSM* task force's press agent. If she asked them for proof of their claim that they were adhering to high standards of scientific research, either they didn't provide it or she didn't convey it to her readers. She simply reported the *DSM* group's claims that "the standards for proposed new categories of mental disorder have been tightened. . . . Nor will categories be added when they are backed by no evidence other than psychiatrists' conviction that they exist" and wrote that Frances and his colleagues had increased "the scientific rigor of the diagnostic process." As with every other example I give in this chapter, the reporter did this despite my having given her abundant evidence that the above claims were dead wrong.

Similarly, a *Newsweek* story included the reporters' assertion that the *DSM* people had carried out "a serious exploration and review of the whole field of PMS," and a Canadian newspaper reporter unquestioningly reported Gold's claim that "the new definition [of PMDD] as a depressive illness is based on science, not politics." In the American Psychological Association's newspaper, the *Monitor*, Tori deAngelis presented PMDD supporters' and opponents' competing claims about the quality of its scientific basis, but she did not write that Gold's own group had concluded in their literature review that the research was preliminary and seriously flawed. Similarly, although deAngelis reported the Gallant study, she did not mention that it demonstrated that the entire construct of LLPDD/PMDD was invalid, because one could not even use it to tell men's symptom checklists from those of women who supposedly fit the PMDD criteria. Although many reporters wrote about PMDD in a way that reified it, that made it seem as though it absolutely does exist, the *Newsweek* coverage included perhaps the most egregious example: "a task force of the American Psychiatric Association has concluded that women with severe PMS actually have a psychiatric disorder." That same article provided a typical example of the way that many reporters wrote as though there were only two possible options: to ignore women when they say they are suffering or to classify them as mentally ill. Such seasoned reporters would surely never have thought to imply that there were only two choices for, say, mourning: to ignore the sorrow of people whose loved ones have died or to say that their mourning is proof that they have a psychiatric disorder. More subtle uses of loaded language were deAngelis's use of the terms "feminist grounds" and "scientific grounds" when describing people's reasons for opposing PMDD as though they were quite separate and *San Francisco Examiner* reporter Carol Ness's phrase that "Caplan contends" that the research is preliminary and flawed. Unless Ness had gone on to note that I had provided solid documentation for my contention (and that it was from Gold's own report, no less!), the word *contends* implies that the contention may be unfounded. Furthermore, Ness did not use similar language to refer to the PMDD supporters' claims, which were indeed unfounded. In his article in the *Kitchener-Waterloo Record*, Miles Socha quoted Gold as saying that the protest was based on misinformation but apparently did not ask for evidence of this before giving Gold's accusation space in his article. Marilyn Linton of the *Toronto Sun* ignored virtually all of the substantive issues and portrayed the matter in the terms of a catfight, saying that "the *fight*" between Paula Caplan and Judith Gold seemed "*strange*" (my italics).

A particularly disturbing misuse of language was Betsy Lehman's report in the *Boston Globe* that I was "threatening to sue" members of the APA and Paula Span's claim in the *Washington Post* that a coalition I had organized had sent the APA a "not-even-slightly-veiled threat [of] lawsuits." Although our letter to the APA Legislative Assembly had certainly included a great deal of information about the basis for lawsuits, it could more accurately have been described as "informing," "explaining," or even "warning" about lawsuits. Since Span had also said that I had resigned from the PMDD work group when "[I] felt [my] counsel was being ignored," I asked Span to print a retraction of both errors. I explained that in the letter to the APA Legislative Assembly, we did not threaten to sue but instead described the grounds on which lawsuits could be based. I also reminded her that I had referred her to a published paper in which I explained that I had resigned because of my concerns about the biased and unscientific nature of the *DSM* process. Eight days after the initial article appeared, the *Post* printed what it called a "clarification":

> [Caplan's letter to the APA] contained a warning that the APA and individual psychiatrists were likely to face lawsuits from female patients and women's groups if it classified PMDD as a mental disorder. In addition, Caplan's resignation from an advisory panel to an APA working group reflected her belief that the group was not proceeding on a scientific basis.

I suspect that many people who read the initial article missed the correction, and in any case, its wording simply added a true report to the previously published false one.

In a very serious omission, many reporters conveyed the APA representatives' claims that no woman had ever been harmed by the label but failed to present any of the ample documentation of such harm that I had provided to them. Lindsay Scotton in the *Toronto Star* conveyed Gold's curious claim that her group had found no *criminal cases* in which a woman had been harmed by use of the diagnostic label, but she failed to mention that our concern was with how it would be used in such *civil cases* as child custody and employment disputes. In Betsy Lehman's otherwise generally well-done *Boston Globe* story, either Lehman or her editor displayed a box on the first page that gave the truly astonishing impression that the main effect of classifying a form of PMS as a mental illness would be to classify all non-PMDD women as *not* mentally ill. The box reproduces in large type Gold's claim, "By saying that the vast majority of women who menstruate do not have a mental disorder, I think we're doing people a service." What was Lehman or her editor thinking of? Would they have highlighted a claim that the terrific thing about sending a few people to the electric chair is that we *don't* send everyone else to it?

Paula Span wrote in the *Washington Post* that the "Donahue" show staff gave their show about the topic the "misleading" title "Psychiatrists Want to Classify Women with PMS as Crazy." I don't know what she thought was misleading about that; it is disingenuous and irresponsible hair-splitting to claim that, although many laypeople equate mental illness with craziness and many people have maliciously hurled accusations about insanity at women who were assumed to have PMS or PMDD, most will not make that equation.

And perhaps the voluminous documentation of harm that women have already suffered in this connection slipped

Paula Span's mind, leading her to write that "So far, fears about the consequences of ratifying PMDD as a mental disorder, expressed both within the APA and outside it, seem based more on what *could* happen than on what has. Take the worries about custody suits. Caplan says women have confided to her that rather than risk losing custody by reason of Premenstrual Dysphoric Disorder, they'll stay with abusive husbands." The women who live every day with abusive husbands because they know women with premenstrual problems may be considered crazy would be surprised to hear that nothing bad has happened to them yet. Indeed, since Span is a reporter, it might have occurred to her that the harm these women are suffering is akin to prior restraint on publication of a newspaper story, which most reporters would consider actual, not potential, harm.

I had told all of the interviewers that PMDD was slated to go in the main text as well as the provisional appendix, and indeed that it had been listed in both places since 1987. However, many of them not only neglected to report that easily verifiable fact but actually quoted APA personnel's (in one case, a top APA administrator's) claims that it was *only* going in the appendix and did nothing to call those claims into question.

Many reporters used negatively loaded words to describe PMDD's opponents but not its advocates. These included writing that we were "outraged," without reporting any evidence that the shoddy science justified our position, and saying that we were "threatening to sue" the APA, when what we had actually done was to inform them of the parallels between the PMDD category and such other inadequately supported products as the Dalkon Shield.

Reporters frequently failed to question claims by *DSM*

spokespeople—claims that I had informed them (and documented for them) were unfounded. Here are a few
more examples.

• Reporters conveyed the APA's claim that it is not possible to conduct research on anything that is not included
in the *DSM*. If they had stopped to think, I believe that
most reporters would have realized that an enormous
amount of mental health research is not about categories
in the diagnostic handbook. Furthermore, they might have
realized that Gold had told them outright that more than
four hundred studies had appeared since LLPDD was first
placed in the manual, and still her committee couldn't find
enough good research to enable them to reach a consensus. Why, then, didn't they wonder (or ask) about the
reasons for the big push to keep the label in the book?
And why, if Gold claimed (as she often did to reporters)
to want to encourage research about men's hormonal
changes, wouldn't she and her group be pushing hard to
get *that* category into the manual?

• Reporters ignored the compelling evidence demonstrating that the whole concept of LLPDD/PMDD is not
valid. Even after I had told her about the research proving
its invalidity (done by PMS research experts), Paula Span
wrote that it "remains to be shown" how well PMDD can
be distinguished from other problems. (As noted in Chapter 5, research by Sheryle Gallant and her colleagues had
shown that women who said they had bad PMS, women
who said they had no PMS, and men did not differ in
symptoms on the PMDD checklist.)

• Reporters conveyed the claim that in order to help
women, it is necessary to keep PMDD in the handbook.
Carol Ness, for example, uncritically reported in the *San
Francisco Examiner* the implication that one cannot help
suicidal women without having this diagnosis, when in fact

one could easily diagnose suicidal women under regular categories of depression that are already in the handbook.

• Reporters unquestioningly reported that only a tiny number of women would be affected, although I had given them documentation of APA officials' admission that at least half a million North American women would be affected.

• Reporters missed the point that inclusion of the label in the main text *in any form*, whether with or without the list of criteria, constitutes a danger to women. In the *Village Voice*, Alissa Solomon reported that LLPDD was listed in the provisional appendix of *DSM-III-R* but "according to standard practice" it was mentioned in the main text, too, without the details (criteria) "which would grant it further legitimacy." However, had Solomon questioned this assertion, she would have learned that it is *not* standard practice to list a label in the main text and exclude the criteria (as noted in Chapter 5). Furthermore, to say that leaving the criteria out of the main text decreases the category's legitimacy does not really reflect actual practice; there is absolutely nothing to prevent a psychiatrist or general practitioner or gynecologist from slapping on a label, *whether or not its criteria are given in the main text*, and rare is the professional who hesitates to use a label for that reason.

• Reporters did not convey the point that PMDD is profoundly gender biased. I don't understand how reporters might hear Judith Gold acknowledge that men have hormonally based mood changes, notice that the *DSM* does not pathologize those, and not figure out that this is blatant gender bias. One of the most egregious examples appeared in Chase's otherwise good article; in that story, Chase quoted LLPDD work group member Nada Stotland as saying that men's hormones need to be studied because teenaged boys drive wildly and have accidents, but both Stotland and the reporter ignored the obvious conclusion that both men's and women's hormonally based moods should be included or both should be omitted from the handbook.

• Reporters uncritically conveyed Gold's claim that women "deserve treatment" through being diagnosed as having PMDD but did not report that antidepressants—Gold's only recommended psychiatric treatment—work no better than placebos and have in many cases harmed women. Related to this was reporters' tendency to miss the point that there is no way to ensure that the label will be applied responsibly or accurately, and even that it is hard to know what "accurate" application of a label means when the criteria have no scientific foundation in the first place.

Examples of Good Reporting

As these articles appeared over a period of several months, there were times when I wondered whether the issues were far more complicated than I had thought and whether I had perhaps done a lousy job of explaining them to the reporters. But the appearance, in rapid succession, of two crystal-clear, beautifully thought-out and well-written columns, one by psychologist Carol Tavris in the *Los Angeles Times* and one by journalist Michele Landsberg in the *Toronto Star*, led me to believe that this was not the case. Both columns were free from errors and misunderstandings about the issues, and both reflected genuine and deep comprehension of the concerns. They were so much better than most of the other print articles—with the exception of the excellent pieces by Kristina Stockwood in the *Montreal Mirror* and Gail Vines in Britain's *New Scien-*

tist magazine—that it is worth repeating some of the points they made. Tavris asked, if this diagnosis is about women who have physical and emotional symptoms associated with the menstrual cycle, why is there no diagnosis, say, for "chronic back pain depressive disorder," a physical condition that can make one anxious, irritable, or depressed? Then, depathologizing what some women report feeling, she wrote that some women like having the PMS label available to them because it gives them an excuse to let off steam once a month. "The comparable excuse for men is drinking," she writes. Tavris ends her column by pointing out the double standard involved in even proposing the PMDD category, because it "feeds the prejudice that women's hormones, but not men's, are a cause of mental illness. That's just ancient superstition in pompous new jargon."

Landsberg, early in her column, points out that "just a couple of decades ago, [even] the label [PMS] didn't exist and neither, for most women, did the symptoms" and then remarks that she finds it very odd "that a version of PMS is about to become an official psychiatric illness." Brilliantly and succinctly summarizing the history of the way women's experiences of premenstrual changes have been received, Landsberg wrote, "Women who do experience premenstrual symptoms have been relieved and even elated to have a name for the condition. 'I'm not crazy—it's PMS!' But now that a psychiatric label is about to be created, the syllogism could read: 'I'm not crazy—I have PMS! Therefore I'm crazy.' " She ends by mentioning some of the dangers likely to result from adoption of the label: "a certain amount of reckless labelling by doctors is inevitable, not to mention soaring insurance costs for over-priced, mood-altering drugs."

Some other writers made other important points. In a lengthy article in the *Village Voice*, Alissa Solomon cast the story in historical and sociocultural perspective in order to show that science does not simply involve a pure search for truth in objective, value-free ways. She wrote:

> the psychiatric profession doesn't exactly have a sterling track record when it comes to women or to accounting for the impact of social reality. . . . This is the profession that, in the 19th century, gave us the mental disorder drapetomania: a slave's "uncomfortable urge to run away from slavery." Meanwhile, the medical world has called the natural aging process an "estrogen deficient disease," and even defined small breasts as an illness. Is it really such a surprise to psychiatrists that women would be suspicious of another diagnosis that seems to medicalize and pathologize something as ordinary as menstruation?

Donaldson and Kingwell took a somewhat different approach to the issue of the APA's subjectivity and bias in their op-ed piece in Canada's *Globe and Mail*:

> Dr. Caplan and her associates have been accused of trying, illicitly, to "politicize" the process of mental-illness definition. It is a common complaint, and one that feminists in many disciplines are used to hearing. It is also incoherent. The difference isn't between people who are political and people who aren't. It's between people who admit the personal and institutional biases of human decision-making, and try to deal with them, and those who retreat behind the smokescreens of scientific objectivity.

Radio and Television Programs

Broadcast shows differ more or less from published articles, depending partly on whether they are live or taped. On live broadcasts, interviewees are usually expected to respond to the interviewer's questions, but one can often manage to work in the important points no matter what one is asked. That, in turn, however, depends greatly on the extent to which the interviewer allows one to answer a question fully. When people from both sides of a debate are being interviewed, interviewers vary in the extent to which they make sure to let both people speak to each issue. The reporters and producers for some taped programs can operate much like print reporters, however, in that they have total control over which interviewees' comments they choose to broadcast and what editorializing remarks of their own they include. Depending on the interviewer's inclination to let one speak—or not—the advantage of a live broadcast can be that one gets to say what one wants and even to show concrete evidence. I want to describe some of the ways that the interviewers or producers from the broadcast programs shaped the way the material was presented.

Two of the radio programs in which I participated were live shows, and two were taped. The first live one was on March 2, 1993, on Canada's CBC radio program "As It Happens," and Judith Gold and I were interviewed simultaneously. The woman interviewer did a generally nice job of asking crucial questions and making sure that both Gold and I got the chance to reply. In my experience, radio and television interviewers tend to have gathered, or been given, somewhat less information before they do their shows than print reporters. So I admired her expression of skepticism when Gold tried to justify associating psychiatric disorder with the menstrual cycle but did so in a way that made no sense: The interviewer asked, "Is [the disorder] related to PMS at all?" and Gold replied, "Only in the sense that it occurs premenstrually." To which the interviewer made an exclamation about "what games" Gold seemed to be playing. The interviewer also asked Gold if a lot of empirical research had been done on the "tiny group of women" that Gold claimed would get the PMDD label. However, when Gold failed to answer truthfully and instead said that the task force had based all of its decisions "purely on scientific research," the interviewer did not challenge her. I had told the "As It Happens" researcher that the scientific research did not justify keeping the label in the manual, and I do not know whether or not she conveyed that information to the interviewer.

Toward the end of the segment, the interviewer asked Gold, "What difference does it make when you classify it as a mental illness?" Gold then spoke but in no way answered the question, and the interviewer unfortunately did not point out Gold's failure to answer, nor did she ask the question again. The interviewer took the important step of asking Gold whether her group had examined men's hormonal changes, but when Gold replied that her committee felt that more research should be done about that area, the interviewer did not ask why only women's hormonal changes were being pathologized, nor did she give me a chance to reply to that question.

The second radio show was an interview I did on March 11 with Ruth Koslak, host of a Minnesota phone-in show. Koslak began by expressing her skepticism about the *DSM* task force's inclusion of PMDD, saying she had read about it in *Newsweek* "and couldn't believe it." Later, she pointed out the double standard that was being applied, commenting that "men in general lash out, blame other people, drink, whereas women go inside and say this is all my fault and get depressed." And still later, she asked whether the psychiatrists' motivation was financial: "Is this all about money?"

On May 16, the national CBC radio show "Sunday Morning" included a pre-taped piece with a great deal of commentary by reporter Beth Gaines, who had spoken to a large number of people as she put her story together. In her own voice, Gaines made it clear that the issue was not whether or not some women suffer but rather whether that suffering should be called a mental illness. She took care to inform her listeners about the kinds of harm that concerned PMDD's opponents, about the extent to which women's socialization and upsetting life situations seem to cause the troubles that were being called signs of psychiatric disorder, about the significant improvement that nonpsychiatric "treatments" like self-help groups have produced, and about the objections to the category from the APA's own Committee for Women in Psychiatry.

On the other hand, Gaines reported uncritically the claim that up to 90 percent of all fertile women experience physical or mental symptoms before their periods; conveyed a picture of PMDD opponents as shrill (by uncritically reporting Gold's comment that the APA is not a bunch of womanhaters, which wrongly suggested that we had used such a crass term for the APA); and failed to question Gold's claim that her group's decision had been based on scientific research. This last point was one I had gone over in great detail with Gaines. When Gold implied that her group's decision could not have been bad for women because all of the group members were female, Gaines allowed that comment to stand, unquestioned.

A taped and edited segment by Michele Trudeau broadcast on National Public Radio's "Weekend Edition" on

July 11 was particularly disappointing. Trudeau talked about PMDD as though it had been proven to be a real mental disorder and unquestioningly conveyed supporters' claims that the category—and its association with depression—is based on good scientific research, that the label is necessary to help women get insurance payments for their therapy (when they can already get reimbursed by being diagnosed simply as "Depressed"), and that research has proven that Prozac helps this "condition." Perhaps worst of all was that, in spite of having been informed about many ways that women have been harmed by being considered premenstrually mentally ill, Trudeau used the voice of only one patient to address the issue of harm, and that was a woman who said she had not been stigmatized by receiving that label.

The first television show on which I appeared to talk about PMDD was the March 5 "Donahue" show, on which Judith Gold was also a guest. The show was broadcast live in some cities and taped for later broadcast in others. I had appeared on "Donahue" three times before to discuss other topics, and I had been impressed most of those times by the host's brilliant grasp of the issues and, often, of their nuances. However, this time he allowed the show's focus to drift from its title, which was about declaring a form of PMS a mental illness, to the question of whether some women have troubles each month. Furthermore, as the latter question became the focus, the implication seemed to be that if women suffer, then we *have to* classify that suffering as a psychiatric disorder. Then, although I made a statement at the beginning of the show about the sexist double standard reflected in selectively calling only women's hormonally based mood changes a mental illness, while ignoring men's, Donahue repeatedly focused only on women. And when an audience member suggested that the label would help women because they do suffer, Donahue neither noted that it should not be a choice between getting no help for one's suffering and having to be called mentally ill nor allowed me or anyone else to say that.

Donahue surprised me by letting Gold get away with the illogical claim, "The link [between the mental illness and PMS] is not hormonal. It just happens during that time of the month" and not allowing time for anyone else to object. At one point, he turned to me and said, "So you are arguing for an arresting of the research"; he might have been trying to allow me to explain that I am not opposed to research per se but, coming from Donahue, his comment runs the risk of sticking in people's minds as the last word on PMDD opponents' attitude. On the positive side, Donahue seemed to take special care to point out that women might be harmed by having the PMDD label pinned on them. However, toward the end of the program, he allowed Gold to get away with claiming that women said to have PMDD would not be regarded as crazy, because PMDD is not consistent with the courts' definition of insanity. Surely Donahue is aware of the widespread hurt caused to women by family members, employers, and "friends" who say, "You're really crazy today. Are you PMSing?" not to mention that being diagnosed as having a mental disorder can make one feel ashamed and depressed even if one has not technically been called insane.

The most disappointing moment for me with the show came during a commercial break. Shortly before the break, I had explained that the work of Gold's own group of experts suggested that at least half a million North American women would be given the PMDD label. Gold had denied that, making her usual claim that only a tiny group of women would be so classified. I had then repeated that the figures were based on an official *DSM* publication, and Gold denied it again. At the break, I told a producer I would like to run to the green room to get that publication and hold it up on camera. She refused to allow me to do so. In retrospect, I probably should have unhooked my microphone and gone off to get it anyway, and I regret not having done so. But I am also frustrated because one of the strengths of shows such as Donahue's is that they often allow one to expose such outright lies, and I am puzzled about why they did so little to make it happen that day. I suspect that it has something to do with mass media people's belief that the public cannot understand what the former often refer to as "complicated scientific material," and Donahue actually made a similar remark on that show. However, most television viewers are perfectly capable of understanding what "half a million women" means and of recognizing that the PMDD committee chairperson's repeated denial of what was in her publication sheds important light on her credibility and the integrity of the whole operation. The next time I appeared on camera with Gold, I was ready for her.

On April 10, Gold and I appeared in a taped interview on the CBC television show "Midday." Gold again made her claim about only a tiny number of women being affected by the PMDD diagnosis, I mentioned the figure of 500,000 derived from a *DSM* publication, and she denied it. I then held up to the camera a copy of the publication in question and said that this was the report that contained that information.

In the introduction to the "Midday" segment, the announcer had implied that PMDD opponents were somehow disbelieving some women's reports of suffering before their periods. The interviewer then immediately talked about PMDD in a way that made it seem as though it were indisputably a real phenomenon. When I described some of the ways that women have suffered because of being diagnosed as premenstrually mentally ill, Gold claimed that her committee "went through all sorts of legal documents and case reports, and since the diagnosis was first introduced in 1967, there are no instances in which the diagnosis has been abused." I found this surprising in light of the harm that I had just described. I thought that an interviewer who was on her toes would have asked Gold how she could make her claim, given the information I had provided.

At the very end of the segment, I pointed out that Gold had just remarked that people of both sexes have hormonal cycles but that only women's cycles made them mentally ill. The interviewer allowed Gold's reply to stand as though it were not a sterling example of lousy logic. What Gold said was, "I didn't say that. I didn't say that women's hormones make them mentally ill. I said that men and women are different and that women get into a severe depression that incapacitates them." As the interviewer knew, severe depression is exactly what Gold was calling a mental illness.

The CTV (Canadian Television network) evening news show on April 14 broadcast a segment put together by Avis Favreau, consisting of her voice overs combined with snippets from interviews with several people. She clearly portrayed some of the kinds of harm that the PMDD label can cause and showed that there is no evidence that PMDD is a legitimate construct or that using this label will help women. However, she did allow to stand Gold's implication that the choice is between ignoring women's complaints and calling them mentally ill, and she failed to question Gold's assertion that only "a small group of women" will be affected, although I had given her the five hundred thousand figure and relevant documentation.

Three days after the APA Board gave its final approval for keeping PMDD in the appendix and listing it in the main text as a Depressive Disorder, I appeared live on NBC television's "Today" show with Robert Spitzer. The first two parts of the segment powerfully conveyed the impression that PMDD is a proven mental illness, both through the words of interviewer Katie Couric (who said, "There is a relatively unknown syndrome that afflicts a small number of women that is much more severe than PMS") and through a videotaped interview with a woman who is described as "having" PMDD and who then reports having very serious depressions. However, Couric ignored the woman's comment that she could shut herself up in a room, "close the blinds, and not come out for weeks at a time." A woman who spends weeks at a time feeling so horrible cannot conceivably be said to have a premenstrual disorder, since the premenstrual phase by definition cannot last for weeks.

Couric also allowed to pass Spitzer's illogical assertion that PMDD is not regarded as a hormonal disturbance, that it is a mood and behavior disturbance that is called "premenstrual" because "that is when it occurs." Later, she asked whether it would be a good thing to "recognize this as an illness so the people who suffer from it can be taken seriously and get the help they need." This was another instance of an interviewer implying that the choice is between ignoring women and pathologizing them.

On the "Today" show, however, I did get the chance to say that "this really should properly be called PMS-gate because of the history of lies and distortions that have characterized the whole process. The APA wouldn't dream of trying to classify half a million Black people or gays as mentally ill with no research to support it."

As a group, then, with a few sparkling exceptions, reporters tended to relay to the public, largely unexamined, the APA's position. The combination of the APA's power and the power of the media is daunting, but it would be tragic if, as a society, we were to lie down and let them continue to work their harm.

10

Where's the Harm, and What Will Help?

The Harm

The act of naming is an act of power. Prospective parents who spend months choosing just the right name for an expected infant know this. Whether it is a given name or a label of mental illness, what you call a person helps determine how you and others will feel about that person.

To assign a name is to act as though you are referring to something that exists, something real. When we name a baby, we are naming something real, but often that is not the case when we label an aspect of a person, or an individual's entire personality, mentally ill. Names shape what we look at and what we think we see. A child trusts its parent when the parent says, "What you are looking at is a dog." As adults, we have been too inclined to believe therapists who tell us, "What you are looking at (or what you are) is a mentally ill person with an Adjustment Disorder or a Self-Defeating Personality." We have too rarely asked, "Is there any proof that there is such a thing as a Self-Defeating Personality Disorder or that this person fits that category?" Nor have we asked often enough,

"Will assigning that label to that person do more harm than good?" In my decades as a clinician, I have rarely heard therapists wrestle with that question but have often heard them debate at length into precisely which mental disorder category to slot a patient. As a result, for instance, beginning in the 1940s, millions of parents were taught by pediatricians, psychologists, and psychiatrists that their children had "Minimal Brain Damage or Dysfunction" or MBD. No one ever managed to change these children's brains, but the label did a great deal of damage. Millions of parents spent years looking at their children and thinking disturbing thoughts like "This child has an abnormal brain" rather than "This child is somewhat clumsy or has trouble learning to add and subtract." Children who were said to have MBD but were relatively fortunate may have received some exercises for their clumsiness or some individual help with their arithmetic, but they could have gotten that assistance without being given the MBD title. As "Minimal Brain Dysfunction" is, happily, becoming a less popular phrase, we perhaps can learn from this kind of historical change in naming that we should think about the consequences before slapping on unproductive or hurtful labels.

Suppose that you're feeling sad, scared, or ashamed, and that you seek relief from those feelings. If the intended helper tells you you have a mental illness called Adjustment Disorder (or Depressive Disorder) because you are *still* feeling low even though it's been six months (or two months) since your spouse left you, you get several messages, all of which are likely to be harmful. One is that you are different from most people, because one would have expected you to be over your upset by now. Another is that you "have" a mental disorder that you probably didn't "know" you had. Believing that something was happening to you and you didn't even realize that it was can add to your insecurity and fearfulness. (As shown in the chart in Chapter 2, "abnormality" in our culture is associated with a vast array of stigmata.) How different that feels from being told truthfully, especially by someone you regard as an expert, that many people in your position feel as you do at this point and then being helped to understand more about why you feel so bad, how to cope with those feelings, perhaps how to feel better, and what you might expect later on.

Although most of this book has been about two *DSM* categories that are especially bad for women, some of the other work I have described (particularly in Chapters 6 and 7) reveals the unscientific character of other *DSM* categories and of the handbook as a whole. Understanding the *DSM* process helps sharpen our ability to assess how anyone judges who is normal, whether we do it ourselves—about ourselves or about other people—or whether it is done about us. I hope that awareness of how the world's most powerful psychiatrists decide who is normal will sensitize us all to the ways such judgments are made by and about us in every aspect of our daily lives. I just heard some people who were beginning to learn meditation berating themselves because they couldn't keep their minds clear for the whole meditation sitting. As soon as the teacher told them that that is what happens to most people, they felt less strange and less inadequate. And how much better have I seen sexual abuse survivors fare when, instead of telling them they have Borderline or Multiple Personality Disorder, therapists help them to express their pain (and support them through it), to notice and appreciate the ways they have struggled to cope with the abuse, and to decide how to go on with their lives.

Too many experts, however, do the former instead of the latter, and because we live in a culture where we learn to shy away from questioning or challenging experts, they do untold damage. One cannot stress enough the havoc wrought in people's lives when they are given labels that are unwarranted and unhelpful. As Phil Brown and Elizabeth Cooksey point out, "Assignment of a diagnostic label is sometimes used as the legal basis for provision of social welfare benefits, and often employed in legal matters such as involuntary commitment, the insanity defense, and competence to stand trial. Labeling may also cause difficulties in purchasing health or life insurance, and lead to discrimination in the workplace and educational and military systems."

All mental health professionals should be challenged when they apply potentially damaging or demeaning interpretations and labels to people. Many of the devastating, real-life consequences of diagnostic labeling and mislabeling have been described throughout the book, but let me mention a few more here, because they are so important. I was recently shown a letter from a lawyer to a psychologist that included these remarks: "Dr. X diagnosed my client as suffering from a Personality Disorder. Your opinion is that she is suffering from a Dissociative Disorder. Obviously, the diagnosis and prognosis for recovery would have serious implications for her ability to care for her children in the future." Canadian therapist Maureen Graham has observed that *DSM* categories have had harmful consequences for people seeking employment as well as for those seeking custody of their children. She also notes that "patients have learned to respond to [being given labels from] the *DSM* by changing their self-definition" in negative ways. And her colleague Nayyar Javed reports that "therapists spend an inordinate amount of time undoing the harm done to people's identity and self-respect by these diagnoses."

It is especially tragic that not only are the already disadvantaged and oppressed those most likely to be harmed by *DSM*-style labels but such labels are sometimes used to great advantage by people who are known oppressors or even perpetrators of violence. For instance, a dentist who pleaded guilty to having fondled between one hundred and two hundred young girls and women patients, ones that he says he thought "were susceptible to being touched," has now sued his insurance company, claiming that his "sexual disorder" makes it impossible for him to work as a dentist, so the insurers should give him $5,000 a month in disability payments. Harold Lief, professor emeritus of psychiatry at the University of Pennsylvania, supported this claim, telling the court that the dentist suffered from "frotteurism," a compulsion to touch women's genitals.

One cannot, then, stress enough how important it is to question and challenge what mental health professionals do. They are human beings. Some of them grew up in your neighborhood. Some got lower grades than you did in high school. Some graduated at the bottom of the programs in which they learned to "treat" you, but you will never know that from the certificates on their walls.

In fortifying oneself to question the mental health experts—and I continue to need fortifying, even after so many years, because one always risks being ignored, dismissed, or attacked—I find it helpful to keep clearly in mind some examples of the harm that has been done by experts who have not been as conscientious or as thoughtful as they ought to be. I shall not even discuss here the worst physical abuses, including prescribing electroshock sessions promiscuously and tying up or isolating people who are not dangerous to themselves or others. I shall begin by mentioning a simplistic and dismissive allegation that was made by psychiatrist Bruno Bettelheim:

> In the turbulent 1960s, Bettelheim (1969) told the United States Congress of his findings: student antiwar protesters who charged the University of Chicago with complicity in the war machine had no serious political agenda; they were acting out an unresolved Oedipal conflict by attacking the university as a surrogate father.

Claims like these clouded the vision of people who were trying to understand the antiwar movement but who respected Bettelheim and others like him.

Some people who have heard that I was writing this book have contacted me to say that I should not write it, because they were given *DSM* diagnoses, were put on drugs, and became happier and better able to function. To such people, I say first that I am pleased and moved to hear that their lives are better. But I also say that not everyone diagnosed as, for instance, "Manic Depressive," has responded well to lithium, and I have friends who suffered permanent physical damage, about which they had not been warned, from the drug. There are similar stories about all psychoactive medications. I would never want anyone to be deprived of a chance for happiness, and if diagnoses have paved the way for drug prescriptions or any other kinds of treatments that helped more than they hurt *and* if patients were fully informed about the possible bad effects and about other ways one could try to deal with their problems, then patients and their therapists should be free to try what they agree on (keeping in mind the enormous power differential between most therapists and patients which makes "agreement between equals" a hard goal to reach). Too often, though, the therapist—and certainly the patient—is not very well informed. As a psychologist specializing partly in research methods, I find it hard to keep up with the research about drugs, for instance, but I have learned that it isn't safe to assume that drug companies' claims and popular media reports about medications are true. I know for a fact that many psychiatrists and other physicians recommend that their patients take Prozac, saying something like, "It seems to be a miracle drug. It helps so many people feel less depressed, and it has very few side effects." They may even mention that there have been some reports of Prozac increasing people's depressive or suicidal tendencies. But I have never heard of one of those therapists giving a patient the kind of information that appeared in the American Psychological Association's *Monitor* in April 1994:

> Up to 75 percent of subjects in various studies showed improvements after taking Prozac, but half of those eventually suffered a recurrence of symptoms, said Jerry Rosenbaum, MD, a psychiatrist at Harvard Medical School who studies psychotropic drugs. Thirty percent of subjects placed on a placebo in the study also showed improvements, Rosenbaum said.

A major consequence of the *DSM*'s medicalization of problems in living—recasting so much loneliness, mourning, disempowerment, insecurity, shame, anxiety, and anger as "diseases" or "disorders"—is that the real sources of many of those upsetting feelings are masked. I do believe some people suffer from hearing voices that frighten them. I know that some people hurt or kill others, and I know many people have terribly upsetting feelings. I do not claim to know how to help all such people. Honest therapists will acknowledge both that the causes of each of those kinds of behavior and feelings are enormously varied, and that a great deal is *un*known about their causes and about what to do for those who suffer from them. But it is clear that a great deal of pain is caused—or exacerbated—by social factors that could be changed if our society took more serious and sweeping steps toward eradicating poverty, prejudice, and violence. Even those people who would argue that poverty, prejudice, and violence are inevitable would understand that it makes little sense to call their effects "mental illness" rather than "the consequences of poverty, oppression, and intimidation." In fact, as Albee observes, *DSM*-backed assumptions that mental and emotional problems are caused by biochemical or brain defects mask the damage done by oppressive social arrangements. One way to describe the *DSM* process would be to say that a relatively small number of people take what they regard as deviant or different and then declare those things medical problems, mental disorders.

I suspect that Louise Armstrong is right when she says that feeling daunted by our apparent powerlessness in the face of obvious, massive needs for social changes, we as a society have chosen to think that individual psychotherapy will solve the problems that need solutions. It is easier, then, to think that an abused, harassed, or underpaid woman has Premenstrual Dysphoric Disorder and should take Prozac than to try to help her leave the abuser or find a well-paying job where she will not be harassed. The former is seductive because it is far easier to implement, and we can delude ourselves into thinking we have really done something good for her. A similar need to find quick solutions pervades much of the treatment of Native American and Native Canadian people. As Lilith Finkler writes:

> Native people who drink excessively are labelled as having "psychoactive substance use disorders." The DSM-III-R does note that "There is a higher incidence of inhalant use among minority youth living in depressed areas," but neglects to explain why. Psychiatrists, typically content to focus on the individual, rarely acknowledge the impact of residential schools, the systematic removal of Native children from their families and their placement into white adoptive homes. Broken treaties, the mass sterilization of Native women, the outlawing of spiritual practices all remain invisible in the medical understanding of human behavior.

How many people, I wonder, have been similarly identified as mentally disordered, "identified patients," getting society off the hook by masking deep societal problems such as racism, sexism, ageism, poverty, homophobia, and oppression of people because of their appearance or mental or physical abilities? At one clinic where I worked for several years, we were told we must not try to arrange for the families to find better jobs or receive adequate welfare monies, although that was what many of them needed most. We were only allowed to give them *DSM* labels and suggest certain kinds of "treatment," all of which were within the realm of traditional mental health care, such as individual or group psychotherapy. My heart used to sink on a regular basis, for I knew that no amount of talking therapy would help them, and I felt sick about wasting the time of these beleaguered people.

What Can Help?

My hope for this book is that it will encourage past, current, and potential therapy patients; their friends and family members; and therapists of all kinds to think carefully about the process and the consequences of choosing and assigning diagnostic labels. Awareness of the way the world's most influential handbook of psychiatric diagnosis has been developed can fortify us in our determination to keep our minds clear and our will strong when we need help or seek to help others; for that awareness can assist us in identifying and setting aside unfounded assumptions, prejudices of many sorts, and harmful ideas about psychological problems and help for those problems. Simply knowing what is—and is not—behind impressive-sounding technical language such as that in the *DSM* should make us more comfortable and confident about questioning the claims experts make about what we are really like. My purpose is not to encourage people to disagree automatically with what therapists say but rather to encourage them, as far as possible, to respect and give weight to their own capacity to think about what they need and to judge whether or not the experts are truly helping them. I know that millions of people who describe themselves as "psychiatric survivors" have been harmed in a wide and devastating variety of ways by mental health professionals of all kinds, and I hope that they will find something useful in this documentation of the ways that so many decisions about normality and abnormality are made. The words of psychologist David Randall are pertinent to the issue of judging whether diagnosis and treatment are helping you: "The key question is, 'Does it move [you] on to where [you] should be?' "

Many therapists have helped patients feel and function better, and most therapists can be helpful at least some of the time. But people seeking assistance should know that although "Many people and facilities sincerely strive to help patients . . . , they do so mainly *without* reference to the official diagnostic framework, or with deliberate circumvention of and opposition to official diagnosis." So patients and prospective patients should ask their therapists whether and how they have diagnosed them and how that diagnosis is affecting their approach to them and to their treatment. Responsible, humane therapists will answer these questions.

It is important to remember, too, that not all psychiatrists are bad—indeed, most were not even involved in the development of the *DSM*—and that psychiatrists are not the only problematic therapists. As psychologist George Albee writes, "Unfortunately, psychologists and social workers accepted meekly the DSM-III (and DSM-III-R) diagnostic system. Instead of fighting it as scientifically dishonest and logically defective, they fell on their knees and begged to be included for reimbursement [with a few notable exceptions]. . . . Abnormal psychology textbook writers . . . also yielded and publishers actually boast about up-to-date coverage of DSM-III-R." So it is advisable to be cautious about therapists of all kinds.

Some people who have been bewildered or otherwise hurt by mental health "treatment" have started groups for "psychiatric survivors," and many such survivors have found those groups enormously helpful. They include Support Coalition International, an alliance of twenty-six U.S. and Canadian grassroots advocacy and support groups (contact Judi Chamberlin, 2 Dow Street, West Somerville, MA 02144, or Sally Clay at E-mail address sallyclay@aol.com); the World Institute on Disability (contact Susan Brown in Oakland, CA, at (510) 763–4100); Resistance Against Psychiatry in Canada (contact Dr. Bonnie Burstow at (416) 538–7103); and the National Association for Rights Protection and Advocacy (contact Bill Johnson, c/o Mental Health Association of Minnesota, 2021 East Hennepin Ave., #412, Minneapolis, MN 55413–2726). The superb newspaper *Dendron* (whose editor is the brave David Oaks, P.O. Box 11284, Eugene, OR 97449–3484; telephone (503) 341–0100; E-mail address: chrp@efn.org) is an invaluable, information-packed resource and also publishes detailed updates about local, national, and international survivors' groups and publications.

People who have been harmed by the "Premenstrual" and "Self-Defeating" labels may have benefited some from the organized and very public protests against these categories, although the outcome in the case of the former was less favorable than the protest by homosexuals against the pathologizing of lesbians and gay men. But there have not been such massive protests about most diagnostic categories, and the tireless efforts of survivors' groups are often mocked or dismissed as the ravings of "crazies." Everyone should listen carefully to what these people are saying.

Other kinds of action are currently in the works. In 1993, psychologist Janet Hyde, president of Division 35 (Women) of the American Psychological Association, established a Task Force on Sexism in Diagnosis. The task force is preparing materials about sexism and other kinds of bias in diagnosis for use in programs where psychotherapists and counselors are trained. It is also spreading the word that its members will provide supporting documentation and expert witnesses for women who have been harmed by the use of these diagnoses (not women who say their PMS upsets them but rather women who, for instance, have been discriminated against in various ways because of having been given these labels). The task force is also interested in working with lawyers and judges to explore the ways that women's rights to equal protection under the law (in both the United States and Canada) are infringed when therapists testify as expert witnesses against women, using as the basis of their testimony unsupported theories and poorly done research that is sexist. For instance, some therapists have testified that women who are battered have "brought it on themselves" by either having "Self-Defeating Personality Disorder" or behaving in horrible ways due to their "Late Luteal Phase Dysphoric Disorder." When alternative, nonsexist explanations (such as that they were assaulted by their partners) that are demonstrably valid are ignored by expert witnesses and judges then accept testimony based on sexist principles, it seems to me that that is a case of representatives of the government (the judges) denying women equal protection and equal rights. The task force may be contacted through a task force member (no phone calls, please): Paula Caplan; c/o K. Quina; Department of Psychology; University of Rhode Island; Kingston, RI 02881.

I want to urge all interested people to assemble petitions, write letters to the experts and the media about what worries you, and obtain publicity about the ways that judgments about who is normal affect you. Consumers of mental health services now have the legal right in many places to obtain their files and find out how they have been diagnosed and what their therapists have written about them. Legal Aid services and private lawyers can sometimes be helpful, as can the psychiatric survivors' groups and groups that advocate for people with disabilities and those that work against racism, ageism, homophobia, and so on.

Therapists might consider thinking less about how to classify and label their patients than about such clearly relevant questions as how they are feeling and why, as well as whether or not they are able to care for and take care of themselves and others. Former mental patient Judi Chamberlin says, "People who have been patients know from their own experience that warmth and support . . . were helpful and that being thought of and treated as incompetent were not."

There are encouraging signs even within the realm of psychoanalysis, which has long been split, Janus-like, into its helpful concentration on detailed, careful listening to what patients say and its attitude that therapists know better than patients what is happening to the patients. Psychoanalyst Evelyne Schwaber, for instance, writes about the importance of the analyst's being open to considering how she affects her patient and to hearing the patient's perspective rather than maintaining a position as the only arbiter of truth.

What therapists—as well as family and friends—can also do is to refuse to produce knee-jerk interpretations of people's problems that consist of forcing human suffering into categories like "masochism" or "codependency." Labeling increases the likelihood that therapists—and patients themselves—will force the patient through the often-deforming mold of a diagnosis, thus misunderstanding much about the patient and overlooking the way that therapists' own blind spots and problems shape their views of their patients. Some therapists can combine careful listening to troubled people with a minimum of preconceptions, with what is suspected or known to help people with certain kinds of problems. Although this approach will not lead to the eradication of all psychological problems or pain, it certainly does not hurt and will probably be of some help. Indeed, one would think it would be the sine qua non of all people who claim to serve others, but often, it is not. In fact, some therapists are so dazzled by or preoccupied with the scientific-seeming *DSM*, as well as with various "treatment" techniques, such as drugs, electroshock therapy, and hospitalization, that they replace a caring approach with instant engagement in choosing a diagnosis and medical treatments, rather than combining a caring approach with responsible consideration of the range of possibly helpful options and their dangers.

Therapists need to know how to think "scientifically," which really means knowing how to evaluate properly what has helped whom and when and under what circumstances, and how to show respect and warmth for their patients. There needs to be a balance between being an evaluator of information from research and being a thoughtful, caring listener, between thinking about general issues and about the individual before you who might or might not be helped by your knowledge of the general. The best way to do the scientific thinking would be to conduct careful research on a large scale, taking account of the important complexities of human behavior and need. The *DSM* people have not done that, nor, for the most part, have other mental health professionals and researchers. Much remains a mystery.

The danger is that people will believe that the *DSM* is the solution to the mystery. This is dangerous for a number of reasons, not the least of which is noted by psychiatrist Joel Kovel, who writes that the handbook exists to serve the needs of therapists, not of their patients. Kovel's perceptiveness is illustrated by Allen Frances's statement that *DSM* categories must come from a long clinical tradition (that is, other *therapists* have to regard the problems in question as mental illnesses: see Chapter 6) and from the description in the *DSM* of the aim of producing a document that is acceptable to professionals from various theoretical orientations and in various settings. Kovel opines that this would be no problem if therapists could be counted on to do what is best for their patients, but he argues that this becomes less likely when patients are seen through the objectifying lens of the *DSM*. He goes on to say that as soon as people are given diagnoses of mental disorders, they are "secured into a system of social relations and power." Instead, he suggests, the focus should be on "the person and his/her relation to the world—instead of being located in the false abstraction of mental disorder."

As therapists, we know so little about what helps people in extremis. It seems to me that, as we struggle to find ways to bring people relief from suffering, we at least ought always to be honest about the possible benefits and possible dangers of what we recommend and about the degree to which what we do is based on science, hunches, or a combination of the two.

And what do I wish the *DSM* people themselves would do? Both as individuals and as a profession and a mental health enterprise, I would urge them to admit that their work is not yet very scientific and reflect that in the title of their handbook. Perhaps they could rename the *DSM* something like *A Proposal for Defining and Classifying Emotional Problems*. They might say that much of what they do is more like art and intuition than like science, and they could promise to handle with loving care, thoughtfulness, and honesty the people who seek help from them—and then do it. Of course, there is every reason also to continue to use scientific research to try to find answers. It is not the doing of research that is the problem. It is the doing of inadequate or bad research and then acting as though it is definitive.

In one APA publication there is this claim:

The process of diagnosis begins with the patient interview. Psychiatrists will order or conduct a careful general medical examination of each patient to assess his or her general health. They will request their patients' medical records from other physicians who've treated their patients. They will carefully question their patients about their past history and the symptoms of their disorder, the length of time they've had the symptoms, and their severity. If it seems warranted, the psychiatrist will also specify a period of observation. It is only after this careful assessment process that a psychiatrist will turn to the *DSM-IV*.

Often, steps of that careful process are skipped. Psychiatrists and all mental health professionals know that, for a variety of reasons, we do not always do everything we should do. To know that but to make public statements that cover up our fallibility is dishonest.

Kirk and Kutchins have pointed out that members of the professions enjoy special privileges, such as being allowed to govern themselves, to control who can join their professions and what kind of training they need, and to regulate the practice of their members. "In return" for all of this freedom, professions are supposed to "abide by their codes of ethics, to protect the interests of their clients, to practice in a disinterested manner, and to use their substantial knowledge for the betterment of society." I wish that the American Psychiatric Association would act accordingly.

Much of this book has been about the ways that people's biases cloud their thinking and even, in the best cases, their honorable intentions of helping people who are suffering. No one is without bias—not I, not the *DSM* people, no one. But it has been said that there is good bias, and there is bad bias, the difference being that good bias *promotes* the search for truth, and bad bias *impedes* it. When bad bias is allowed to drive the business of classifying and labeling human beings, it strangles our speech and constricts the space in which we can feel safe, free, and proud.

Appendix A: Newspaper and Magazine Articles about PMDD

1. Goode, Erica. 1992. Sick, or just quirky? Psychiatrists are labeling more and more human behaviors abnormal. *U.S. News and World Report*, February 10, 49–50.

2. Tavris, Carol. 1993. You haven't come very far, baby: Women should be wary when psychiatrists want to label physical symptoms as a new mental disorder. *Los Angeles Times*, March 4, B7.

3. Landsberg, Michele. 1993. Calling PMS a psychiatric disorder is sheer madness. *Toronto Star*, March 12, J1.

4. Seligmann, Jean, with David Gelman. 1993. Is it sadness or madness? Psychiatrists clash over how to classify PMS. *Newsweek*, March 15, 66.

5. Linton, Marilyn. 1993. PMS funding a headache. *Toronto Sun*, March 18, 52.

6. Socha, Miles. 1993. PMS designation as psychiatric illness rapped. Protest grows against "oppressive" labeling of some premenstrual syndrome. *Kitchener-Waterloo Record*, March 25, F8.

7. McMillen, Liz. 1993. Proposal to define premenstrual syndrome as a mental disorder draws fire. *Chronicle of Higher Education*, March 31, A8.

8. Solomon, Alissa. 1993. Girl crazy? Psychiatry tries to make PMS a mental illness. *The Village Voice*, April 6, 32–33.

9. Pelletier, Francine. 1993. Les regles de la folie. *Le Devoir*, April 15.

10. Stockwood, Kristina. 1993. Crazy idea: PMS to be classified as mental illness. *Montreal Mirror*, April 15, 9.

11. Scotton, Lindsay. 1993. PMS debate: Is it a mental disorder? *Toronto Star*, April 27, B1, B3.

12. Suh, Mary. 1993. Severe PMS: Is it mental illness or just normal behavior? *Ms*, May/June.

13. McIver, Mary. 1993. Shrink-wrapped. *Homemaker's*, May, 126.

14. Laurence, Leslie. 1993. Debating classification of PMS. *Connecticut Post*, May 2.

15. Lehman, Betsy. 1993. A little revision is creating a big furor. *Boston Globe*, May 10, A1, A16.

16. Donaldson, Gail, and Mark Kingwell. 1993. Who gets to decide who's normal? *The Globe and Mail*, May 18, A23.

17. Ness, Carol. 1993. Premenstrual moods a mental illness? *San Francisco Examiner*, May 20, A1, A16.

18. Chase, Marilyn. 1993. Version of PMS called disorder by psychiatrists. *Wall Street Journal*, May 28, B1, B3.

19. Feminists assail move to call PMS a disorder. 1993. *News and Leader*, May 30, 10A.

20. Span, Paula. 1993. Vicious cycle: The politics of periods. *Washington Post*, July 8, C1–C2.

21. Grimes, Charlotte. 1993. Psychiatrists are crazy, man. *St. Louis Post–Dispatch*, July 15.

22. Vines, Gail. 1993. Have periods, will seek therapy. *New Scientist*, July 31, 12–13.

23. Cornacchia, Cheryl. 1993. Is PMS a mental illness? *The Gazette*, August 2, A1, F2.

24. deAngelis, Tori. 1993. Controversial diagnosis is voted into latest DSM: Opponents cite potential of harm to women. *American Psychological Association Monitor*, September, 32–33.

25. Segal, Emma F. 1993. The D.S.M. debate. *New Woman*, March, 95.

Appendix B. Broadcast Segments or Shows about LLPDD/PMDD

Radio Shows
March 2, 1993—Interview on CBC radio show "As It Happens"
March 11, 1993—Interview with Ruth Koslak on WCCO radio, Twin Cities, Minnesota
May 16, 1993—Documentary segment by Beth Gaines on CBC radio show "Sunday Morning"
July 11, 1993—Documentary segment by Michelle Trudeau on National Public Radio show "Weekend Edition"

Television Shows
March 5, 1993—"Donahue"
April 10, 1993—CBC television show "Midday"
April 14, 1993—CTV evening news segment with Avis Favreau
July 10, 1993—"Today" show interview with Katie Couric

Notes

p. xi   *"Reading about the evolution"* Armstrong, 1993.

Preface

p. xv   *remarkable books*   Breggin, 1991; Burstow and Weitz, 1988; Chamberlin, 1978; Chesler, 1972; Goffman, 1961; Masson, 1984a, 1984b, 1986, 1988, 1991; Millett, 1991; Penfold and Walker, 1983; and Rush, 1980.

p. xvi   *interested readers*   Laidlaw, Malmo, and Associates, 1990; Robbins and Siegel, 1983; Siegel and Cole, 1991; Siegel, 1988; Jordan et al., 1991; Schwaber, 1983; Chrisler and Howard, 1992.

p. xvi   *Thomas Szasz*   Szasz, 1961.

p. xvii   *R. Walter Heinrichs*   Heinrichs, 1993, p. 230.

p. xvii   *When responsible reviews of research*   See also Breggin, 1991; Penfold and Walker, 1983; Chesler, 1972; Caplan, 1987; and Caplan, 1991a.

p. xvii   *environmental allergies*   For example, see King, 1988; O'Shea and Porter, 1981.

p. xvii   *As psychologist Carol Tavris*   Tavris, 1992, p. 178.

p. xviii   *"Like all semireligious"*   Advertisement, 1986.

p. xix   *Although increasing numbers*   For example, see Caplan, 1994b.

p. xix   *The 1987 edition*   APA, 1993b, p. 2.

p. xix   *Related products*   Kirk and Kutchins, 1992, p. 197.

p. xx   *In fact*   Kirk and Kutchins, 1992, p. 194.

p. xx   *the number of psychiatrists*   Kirk and Kutchins, 1992, p. 8; Goleman, 1990; Schulberg and Manderscheid, 1989.

p. xx   *In all*   Span, 1993.

p. xx   *I believe that*   Caplan, 1992.

p. xxi   *As Jerome Frank*   Frank, 1949, p. 36.

p. xxii   *Laypeople generally*   see Caplan, 1994b.

p. xxii   *As I have written*   Caplan, 1994b.

p. xxiii   *Carol Mithers*   Mithers, 1994, p. 10.

p. xxiii   *Therapy has been defined*   Raimy, 1950, p. 3.

p. xxiii   *Hans Strupp*   Strupp, 1986, p. 121.

p. xxiii   *Judi Chamberlin*   Chamberlin, 1978, pp. 9–10.

p. xxiii   *By now, more than two decades*   e.g., Caplan and Caplan, 1994; Caplan, 1994b.

Chapter 1

p. 1   *Martha Minow*   Minow, 1987, p. 1901.

p. 1   *Peter Breggin*   Breggin, 1991, p. 141.

p. 6   *What does it say*   Miller, 1994, p. B1.

p. 6   *And this study*   Kessler, McGonagle, Zhao, Nelson, Hughes, Eshleman, Wittchen, and Kendler, 1994.

p. 7   *In 1984*   Caplan, 1984.

p. 8   *Diagnostic and Statistical Manual*   APA, 1987.

p. 8   *1994 edition*   APA, 1994a.

p. 9   *Some people*   e.g., see Millett, 1991; Breggin, 1991; and others such as Chamberlin, 1978.

p. 10   *their lengthy report*   Gold et al., 1993.

p. 11   *The professionals most concerned*   APA, August 1993, p. 1.

p. 13   *I firmly believe*   Caplan, 1992.

p. 14   *"I had been in therapy . . ."*   Caplan, 1994a.

p. 14   *In fact, some*   Waxler, 1977, 1979, cited by Marshall, 1982, p. 176.

p. 15   *"It was through the development . . ."*   Kirk and Kutchins, 1992, p. 75.

p. 16   *a recent study of patients*   Harris, Hilton, and Rice, 1993.

p. 18   *Halcion*   This negative effect and others from Halcion have been documented even more widely in recent years.

p. 20   *Psychiatrist Peter Breggin*   Breggin, 1991, p. 235.

p. 20   *"problems in living"*   Szasz, 1961.

p. 24   *After all, it is widely*   Caplan, 1992.

p. 24   *However, as will be*   APA, 1994a, p. xxi.

p. 24   *the DSM authors*   APA, August 1993, p. 3.

p. 25   *It is now well known*   see Masson, 1984; Rush, 1980.

p. 25   *As Jeffrey Moussaieff Masson*   Masson, 1984b.

p. 25   *Of the thousands*   Masson, personal communication, January 2, 1994.

p. 26   *Yet despite all of this*   APA, August 1992, p. 1.

p. 27   *Furthermore, although the DSM authors*   APA, August 1993, p. 1.

p. 28   *Peter Breggin*   Breggin, 1991, p. 344.

p. 28   *The New Harvard*   Nicholi, 1988.

p. 28   *"contains the official . . ."*   Kirk and Kutchins, 1992, p. 12.

p. 29   *"By developing . . ."*   Kirk and Kutchins, 1992, p. 14.

p. 30   *55 percent of clinical social workers*   Kutchins and Kirk, 1988, Kirk and Kutchins, 1988.

p. 30   *"Unfortunately, since psychiatry dominates . . ."*   Kutchins and Kirk, 1988a, 1988b.

p. 31   *racialized people*   Many people who have been called "people of color," "members of minority groups," or "non-whites" have expressed their dislike of those terms. Nayyar Javed drew my attention to the term "racialized," which reflects the fact that the division of people into races is a sociopolitical act that is wrongly assumed to be scientifically justified.

Chapter 2

p. 33 *"Some critics wonder ..."* Goode, 1992, p. 49.

p. 33 *Mental health researchers* see Kirk and Kutchins, 1992, pp. 133ff., and this volume, Chapter 6.

p. 36 *What do we make* Marshall, 1982, pp. 34–35.

p. 37 *"whatever leads people to seek psychotherapy"* Harris, Birley, and Fulford, 1993.

p. 37 *as a result of seeking* Finkler, 1993.

p. 37 *After first announcing* see Rush, 1980; Masson, 1984, for discussion of this sequence of events.

p. 39 *With her groundbreaking book* Chesler, 1972.

p. 39 *which diagnostic labels* Desmond, cited by Marshall, 1982.

p. 39 *racial stereotypes* Loring and Powell, 1988.

p. 39 *stereotypes about different ways* Desmond, cited by Marshall, 1982; Loring and Powell, 1988; Rosenfield, 1982; Broverman et al., 1970.

p. 40 *stereotypes about how people* Marks, Seeman, and Haller, 1974.

p. 40 *the socioeconomic class* Marshall, 1982; Haney 1969, 1970, cited by Marshall, 1982; Hollingshead and Redlich, 1958.

p. 40 *the kind of training* DeWolfe, 1974, and Temerlin, 1968, both cited by Marshall, 1982.

p. 40 *the therapist's internal response* Light, 1980.

p. 40 *the interaction* Rosenberg, 1984.

p. 40 *whether or not the patient* Murray, 1978, cited by Marshall, 1982.

p. 40 *Hundreds of years ago* Marshall, 1982, p. 27.

p. 40 *Later, in the name of religion* Ibid., p. 28.

p. 41 *What has been shown* e.g., Laidlaw, Malmo, and Associates, 1990; Rawlings and Carter, 1977; Umbarger, Morrison, Dalsimer, and Breggin, 1962; Luborsky, Crits-Christoph, Mintz, and Auerback, 1988.

p. 41 *"the notion of mental illness ..."* Szasz, 1961, p. 205.

p. 41 *"How could ..."* Armstrong, 1993, p. 133.

p. 41 *"some harm is ..."* Johnson, 1993.

p. 43 *And mental health* Random House Webster's College Dictionary.

p. 44 *One could divide* Offer and Sabshin (1966) have suggested a slightly different set of models, i.e., normality as health or as utopia (somewhat parallel to my model of absence of conflict or anxiety), as being average (parallel to my infrequency model), or as consisting of a particular process over time.

p. 46 *the average family* Kazak et al., 1989.

p. 48 *By this standard* J. B. Miller, 1984.

p. 48 *To use this kind of approach* see, for example, Caplan and Caplan, 1994.

p. 49 *only males were observed* see Caplan and Caplan, 1994; Gilligan, 1982, for critiques.

p. 50 *In a famous 1970 study* Broverman, Broverman, Clarkson, Rosencrantz, and Vogel, 1970.

p. 52 *"To be mentally ill . . ."* Dumont, 1994, p. 63.

p. 53 *The terms* normal *and* abnormal APA, 1980.

p. 53 *"no assumption that each category"* APA, 1994a, p. xxii.

p. 53 *If the* DSM *authors* Carson, 1994. Psychologist Robert Carson has said that "probably the most fundamental of the several serious problems of the [*DSM*] has been the inability or unwillingness of institutionalized psychiatry to renounce in explicit fashion the firmly bounded categorical format. . . . I can only presume that the reason for this . . . has somehow to do with the perceived need to maintain the medical science disease metaphor. My own view is that a psychiatry aspiring to be a science cannot afford self-deception of this magnitude" (1994, p. 5). He notes that discrete, non-overlapping categories of people's behavior are unnatural: ". . . nature seems to abhor discrete, discontinuous categories almost as much as it was once said to abhor vacuums" (p. 2). Acknowledging that this makes it difficult to come up with a diagnostic system, he then opines that "in the long run we shall do better to face up to and accept it as a significant coping challenge, rather than engage on the one hand in endlessly quixotic pursuits or on the other in denial and implicit claims of a precision we do not have and cannot get. The latter course, an especially common one, leads to the sorts of confusions and peculiarities we routinely observe in clinical personality diagnosis . . ." (p. 3). Carson also criticizes the *DSM* on the grounds that so little attention is paid therein to interpersonal behavior, which he describes as "the ultimate, defining medium in which personality is manifested. . . . In fact, some of us continue to entertain fantasies of overthrowing the DSM in favor of a taxonomic model that is distinctly interpersonal in focus, and hence more consonant with the real problems of real people" (pp. 2, 4).

p. 53 *Apparently, in 1975* Armstrong, 1993, p. 134.

p. 54 *"Mental disorders are a subset . . ."* Ibid., p. 135.

p. 54 *As Louise Armstrong* Ibid., p. 169.

p. 54 "a clinically significant . . ." APA, 1994a, pp. xxi–xxii.

p. 56 *homosexuality* It does not appear to be listed any longer in the *DSM-IV,* as far as I could tell, although therapists could choose to include it under the headings of "Sexual Dysfunction Not Otherwise Specified" or "Paraphilias Not Otherwise Specified."

p. 56 *The APA's vote* Girard and Collett, 1983.

p. 56 *The one potentially good aspect* APA, 1994a.

p. 58 *"The question What is mental illness? . . ."* Chamberlin, 1978, p. 10.

Chapter 3

p. 59 *"The history of mental health care . . ."* Marshall, 1982, p. 23.

p. 59 *"a normal family . . ."* Walsh, 1982, described by Kazak et al., 1989, p. 278.

p. 60 *As mentioned* Chesler, 1972; Desmond, cited by Marshall, 1982; Loring and Powell, 1988; Rosenfield, 1982; Broverman et al., 1970; Marks, Seeman, and Haller, 1974; Marshall, 1982; Haney 1969, 1970, cited by Marshall, 1982; Hollingshead and Redlich, 1958; Rosenberg, 1984; Murray, 1978, cited by Marshall, 1982. Indeed, it is a sign of the pervasiveness of bias and prejudice of all kinds among the population of therapists that the American *Psychological* Association found it necessary to develop guidelines for therapists and counselors to help them avoid sexist, heterosexist, homophobic, ageist, racist, and other ethnically biased remarks and behavior (Gartrell, 1994; Guidelines for providers, 1993; Schaie, 1993; Rothblum et al., 1986; Denmark, Russo, Frieze, and Sechzer, 1988).

p. 61 *New Harvard Guide* Nicholi, 1988.

p. 61 *I noticed years ago* Caplan, 1994b.

p. 61 *these brief dialogues* Shepard and Lee, 1970, pp. 54–55.

p. 62 *a massive DSM-IV* APA, 1994a. The 374 diagnoses include twenty-six under the more inclusive heading of "V Codes— Other Conditions That May be a Focus of Clinical Attention." In the *DSM-III-R*, the heading had been the less pathologizing "V Codes—Conditions *Not Attributable to a Mental Disorder* That Are a Focus of Attention or Treatment" (my italics).

p. 62   *"There is little agreement ..."* Kirk and Kutchins, 1992, p. 226.

p. 62   *When there is no clear demarcation* The *DSM* people say there is no clear distinction between what is and what is not a mental disorder, which leads one to wonder how they can have a whole book of details allegedly advising exactly how to recognize specific kinds of mental disorders in some cases (e.g., the symptoms must be of at least one week's duration) but blithely leaving it up to each individual clinician to decide who is and is not "markedly angry," for instance? If the *DSM* authors do not believe there is such a thing as mental disorder, they should not claim to be able to make fine distinctions among the varieties of this nonexistent entity. If they do believe in it, it seems that their claim that mental disorders are not discrete entities would appear to be a disingenuous attempt to ward off their critics.

p. 62   *Ben Carniol* Carniol, 1987.

p. 63   *Experience with women survivors* Cole and Barney, 1987; Levene, 1992.

p. 63   *When the latter approach* Cole and Barney, 1987.

p. 64   *Maurice Temerlin* Temerlin and Trousdale, 1969.

p. 64   *problems in living* Szasz, 1961, 1970.

p. 65   *The psychologist who showed* Temerlin and Trousdale, 1969, p. 25.

p. 66   *"Simply state ..."* Ibid., p. 25.

p. 66   *"looked like a normal ..."* Ibid., p. 25.

p. 67   *A similar outcome* Williams, Gibbon, First, Spitzer, Davies, Borus, Howes, Kane, Pope, Rounsaville, and Wittchen, 1992.

p. 68   *Susie Orbach* Orbach, 1990.

p. 68   *Szasz has said* Szasz, 1961, p. 75.

p. 69   *J. L. T. Birley* Harris, Birley, and Fulford, 1993.

p. 69   *"it incorrectly implied ..."* APA, August 1993, p. 4.

p. 69   *Judi Chamberlin* Chamberlin, 1978.

p. 69   *can also cause depression* Breggin, 1991.

p. 70   *the patient's father* Caplan, 1989a.

p. 70   *Even what may seem truly bizarre* e.g., Caplan, 1987.

p. 71   *George Orwell* Orwell, 1977.

p. 71   *Robert Butler's* Butler, 1975.

p. 71 *A related manifestation* Siegel, 1993.
p. 72 *Patterns similar to that with respect to aging* For instance, psychologist Doris DeHardt has described the way that many marriage therapists perpetuate the sexist power distribution that frequently obtains in families, encouraging the men to behave in more dominant ways and the women in less dominant ones: DeHardt, 1992.
p. 72 *Today it is possible* Albee, 1990.
p. 72 *"How many complaints . . ."* Marcus, 1991, p. 63.
p. 73 *One might take the view* Caplan, 1992.
p. 73 *Consciousness-raising* see Steinem, 1992.
p. 73 *Rachel Perkins* Perkins, 1991.
p. 74 *Wendy Kaminer's* Kaminer, 1992.
p. 75 *Schofield* Schofield, 1964.
p. 75 *"A human failing"* Breggin, 1991, p. 39.
p. 76 *Psychiatrist Gerald Klerman* Klerman, in Nicholi, 1988, p. 75.
p. 77 *Kirk and Kutchins* Kirk and Kutchins, 1992, p. 221.
p. 77 *Journalist Erica Goode* Goode, 1992, p. 50.
p. 78 *To receive the diagnosis* APA, 1994a, p. 498.
p. 78 *Because Hypoactive Sexual Desire Disorder* APA, 1994a , e.g., p. 498.
p. 79 *If they are reserved* Caplan, 1981.
p. 79 *I pointed out* e.g., Caplan, 1987; Lenore Walker, 1987; Brown, 1986; Rosewater, 1987.
p. 80 *very high frequency* Caplan and Hall-McCorquodale, 1985a; 1985b.
p. 80 *Robert Pepper-Smith* Pepper-Smith and Harvey, 1990.
p. 81 *In the past twenty five years* Kirk and Kutchins, 1992, pp. 213–14.
p. 82 *As I write, the current issue* Kessler, McGonagle, Zhao, Nelson, Hughes, Eshleman, Wittchen, and Kendler, 1994.

Chapter 4
p. 83 *"One should be able . . ."* B. Walker, 1987, p. 4.
p. 83 *If you pictured* See also Faludi, 1991, esp. p. 361.
p. 85 *Mark Zimmerman* Zimmerman, 1988, p. 1137.
p. 85 *In fact, the DSM* Larkin and Caplan, 1992.
p. 89 *At November's Ad Hoc Committee meeting* Walker, 1986.
p. 89 *"had voted to invest . . ."* Caplan, 1987, p. 257.
p. 90 *"using such a diagnosis . . ."* Rosewater, 1985, p. 1.
p. 90 *"To psychologist Renee Garfinkel . . ."* Leo, 1985, p. 76.
p. 90 *In response to this* Spitzer, December 30, 1985, p. 7.
p. 91 *"[T]hey were having a discussion . . ."* Faludi, 1991, p. 361.

p. 92 *"Whatever is, is right"* Pope, 1733/1962.

p. 93 *The Myth of Women's Masochism* Caplan, 1985.

p. 94 *Furthermore, none* Spitzer, 1985, p. 2.

p. 94 *This withholding* see also Kirk and Kutchins, 1992, for a detailed account of this practice.

p. 97 *"the Surgeon General . . ."* Carmen, 1985, p. 7.

p. 97 *Lenore Walker's report* L. Walker, 1986.

p. 97 *"The American Psychological Association . . ."* APA's Council of Representatives, February 2, 1986, statement.

p. 98 *a collective of women mental health professionals* They included Teresa Bernardez, Laura Brown, Joan Cummerton, Renee Garfinkel, Barbara Hart, Beverly McGain, Virginia O'Leary, Lynne Rosewater, Adrienne Smith, Judy Sprei, and Lenore Walker.

p. 100 *Jean Baker Miller* According to Kutchins and Kirk (in press, Chapter XX, Part I, p. 27), Spitzer had asked Teresa Bernardez, who was then head of the APA's Committee on Women, to suggest someone to speak against SDPD. They write that "Bernardez did not merely suggest both Jean Baker Miller and Paula Caplan as possible speakers, she herself invited them to make presentations. Spitzer, as organizer of the symposium, was clearly miffed that she did not follow his instructions, reminded Bernardez that she did not have the authority to appoint the speakers at his meeting, and told her that if she wanted her own symposium, she should organize one [Letter Spitzer to Bernardez, October 31, 1985]." I only learned about that in May 1994, when I read the Kutchins and Kirk manuscript.

p. 102 *"Nine Problems . . ."* see Caplan, 1987, Afterword chapter for discussion of all of these nine problems.

p. 102 *I said that each year* Caplan, May 13, 1986.

p. 103 *Author Louise Armstrong* Armstrong, 1993, p. 152.

p. 104 *It is relevant to note here* APA, 1980, p. 6.

p. 104 *"The criteria . . ."* Committee on Women, 1985.

p. 105 *Rosewater refers* Rosewater, 1987.

p. 109 *In December 1986* Caplan, 1986.

p. 110 *"without mentioning the controversy . . ."* Breggin, 1991, p. 335.

p. 110 *fewer than two hundred people* In the *DSM-IV*, rather than listing the core members of each committee, the authors chose to print lengthy lists of "Advisers," which included both core members and people who, like me, had been asked to serve as "consultants or advisors." Many of the names they listed belonged to people who had strongly objected to what ultimately went into the manual or who had never been consulted, but this padding enhances the appearance of having a large and broadly based group of participant contributors. Even so, white male psychiatrists still account for the majority of names on those lists, and those with the decision-making power almost exclusively fit that category.

p. 110 *Gerald Klerman wrote* Nicholi, 1988, p. 77.
p. 111 *a memo from Dr. Frances* Frances, 1988, p. 1.
p. 112 *The Myth of Women's Masochism* Caplan, 1987.
p. 112 *In May, having heard nothing* Caplan, 1989d.
p. 112 *She promised* Fiester, 1989a, p. 3.
p. 113 *the "importance of examining . . ."* Fiester, 1989a, p. 1.
p. 113 *"careful scrutiny"* Ibid., p. 2.
p. 113 *"Unfortunately, it arrived . . ."* Gunderson, 1989a, p. 1.
p. 113 *"The ultimate fate . . ."* Ibid., p. 1.
p. 114 *In fact, there is virtually* Caplan and Gans, 1991; Herman, 1988.
p. 114 *Frances wrote on October 26* Frances, 1989a, p. 1.
p. 114 *"a bit too polemical"* Ibid.
p. 114 *Having thus been urged* Caplan, 1989c, p. 1.
p. 114 *"I was not surprised . . ."* Caplan, 1989d, p. 1.
p. 115 *"was an important source . . ."* Gunderson, 1989b, p. 1.
p. 115 *And in fact, the minutes he sent me* Minutes, 1989.
p. 115 *On November 17* Fiester, 1989b.
p. 115 *With the review* Fiester, 1989b.
p. 115 *I read her paper* Caplan, 1989d.
p. 116 *"I had very little time . . ."* Caplan, 1989d, p. 1.
p. 116 *Gans and I submitted our review* Caplan and Gans, 1991.
p. 117 *After removing every word* Caplan, 1989b.
p. 118 *"DSM-III reflects . . ."* APA, 1980, p. 1.
p. 118 *"consistency with data . . ."* Ibid., p. 2.
p. 118 *"I think we differ . . ."* Frances, 1990a, p. 1.
p. 119 *"SDPD—Dr. Frances mentioned . . ."* Minutes, 1990.
p. 119 *On November 8, 1990* Caplan, 1990a.
p. 120 *Dr. Margaret Jensvold* Jensvold, personal communication, May 23, 1994.
p. 121 *"Tailhook of the Medical Establishment"* Jensvold and Breggin, 1992.

Chapter 5
p. 122 *"come to some conclusion . . ."* Gold, February 10, 1989, p. 1.

p. 123 *wrote a review of it*   Caplan, McCurdy-Myers, and Gans, 1992a.

p. 124 *Table 1*   from APA, 1987.

p. 126 *custody proceedings* "The court in Tingen v. Tingen, 446 P. 2d (Or. 1968), allowed incidence of PMS to be considered as one of the factors in determining the best interest of the child": Solomon, 1995.

p. 127 *at least five hundred thousand women*   I had arrived at this estimate in as conservative a fashion as possible, using the *DSM* Task Force's own numbers from their *DSM Update* of January/February 1993. If the population of the United States is rounded off at 250,000,000, one can estimate the number of females by multiplying that figure by 52 percent, because females account for about 52 percent of the nation's people, and that multiplication gives a figure of 130,000,000. Underestimating, if anything, I then assumed that only half of that number—65,000,000—are women who are neither premenarcheal nor postmenopausal. Next, I multiplied that last figure by 3 percent, using the task force's claim that only 3 percent of women of menstruating age complain of having PMS (others have put that figure much higher), and reached a figure of 1,950,000 women. Next, I multiplied 1,950,000 by 14 percent, the LLPDD committee's lowest estimate of the proportion of women complaining of PMS *who would receive the LLPDD diagnosis*, and got a figure of 273,000 women. If, instead of the committee's lowest estimate of 14 percent one uses the committee's highest estimate of 45 percent, one gets a figure of 877,500. I then chose the figure of 500,000 as being partway between the 14 percent and 45 percent figures but clearly a low estimate, if anything.

p. 127 DSM-IV Update   APA, 1993a.

p. 128 *no hormonal link*   Reame, Marshall, and Kelch (1992), for instance, found from their four-year study of four key hormones including progesterone that there were no hormonal differences between women with and women without PMS symptoms. Hamilton and Gallant (1993) report that progesterone treatments for symptoms described as premenstrual are ineffective. Schmidt et al. (1991) manipulated women's actual endocrine environment, so that the women they studied believed themselves to be premenstrual but actually were in the hormonal state women experience postmenstrually. In that state, these women reported experiencing their usual, premenstrual-like symptoms, suggesting that beliefs about one's hormonal state have more effect on one's experience of symptoms than does one's actual hormonal condition.

p. 128 *men have mood cycles* see Steinem, 1992; Parlee, 1978a; and Tavris, 1992, for descriptions of some of the relevant research. Here, I shall give just a few examples of this work. Parlee (1978a) cites twelve studies showing that adult males have hormonal cycles and cycles of moods and notes that there are "significant infradian rhythms in the feelings, moods, and activation levels of adult men" (p. 10). Rossi (1974) has found clearer evidence of weekly mood cycles in men than in women. Houser (1979) measured levels of testosterone and other hormones in men's blood and gave them mood questionnaires, behavioral measures (e.g., of reaction time and arm-hand steadiness), and the widely used Menstrual Distress Questionnaire (omitting its title and the item "painful breasts"). She found significant relationships between the men's hormone levels and their moods, including decreases in their good humor and the steadiness of their hands as their plasma testosterone increased. And in a large study of 4,462 male veterans, psychologists James Dabbs and Robin Morris (1990) found a relationship between high testosterone and delinquency, drug use, having many sex partners, conduct disorders, abusiveness, and violence. As Tavris points out, these are correlational data, showing only a connection rather than the direction of a cause-effect relationship, and some kinds of behavior can raise testosterone level, as well as the reverse. However, cause-effect relationships between hormones and behavior in women can also go in both directions, a point that is rarely made in discussions of "PMS."

p. 128 *Gloria Steinem* Steinem, 1994, p. 51.

p. 128 *Even Gold* Gold et al., 1993.

p. 129 *They explicitly questioned* Gold et al., 1993, p. 68.

p. 129 *In fact, a recent New York Times* Lavin, 1994.

p. 129 *In an interview* Cornacchia, 1993.

p. 129 *Dianne Corlett* Corlett, 1993.

p. 130 *Grimes reported* Grimes, 1993.

p. 130 *"women with PMDD . . ."* deAngelis, 1993, p. 33.

p. 130 *"Women are being given . . ."* Vines, 1993, p. 13; see also Peter Breggin, 1991, who reports that, although antidepressants are given to help prevent suicide, there is no published evidence that the antidepressants are helpful in reducing suicide, and Avery and Winokur's 1976 study actually shows an *increased* suicide rate among patients receiving antidepressant therapy. Breggin also reports that antidepressants can well *cause* depression.

p. 131 *"Some members of the [LLPDD] committee ..."* Frances, March 12, 1993.

p. 131 *"help women who* think ..." Pincus, 1993.

p. 131 *The PMSgate stories* Mack, 1994. Mack's clear allegiance to the *DSM* group is reflected in such press release–type statements (in what is presented as a scholarly document) as: "DSM-IV [his uncle's edition of the manual] was a landmark in itself, because, unlike most decisions in DSM-III and DSM-III-R, a careful process of empirical review would provide data to answer all questions the manual faced, including the questions over PMDD and SDPD" (p. 84). Chapters 4, 5, 6, and 7 of this book demonstrate the falsity of that claim, as many others have done, and I had made all of that supporting documentation available to Mack.

In his thesis, Mack kept restating the claim that there was nothing political about the *DSM* people's handling of the controversies over homosexuality, SDPD, and LLPDD. The core of his argument was that all of their decisions were driven by the need to "remedicalize" the manual, and for some reason he did not explain, he equated "remedicalization" with choosing categories that could be empirically analyzed. The poor quality of his reasoning is reflected, for instance, in his claim that this remedicalization was the reason that "Homosexuality" was removed from the manual and replaced by "Ego Dystonic Homosexuality" and "Sexual Orientation Disturbance" although the two latter labels are no more empirically analyzable than the former. Mack's choice of language and his penchant for ignoring or distorting the facts were also characteristic of the *DSM* group itself. He falsely claimed that I had said that "the" agenda of the APA was the continuing mistreatment of women (p. 73), when I have neither thought nor said that that was its agenda. He also claimed that "Feminists would misleadingly portray [SDPD and LLPDD] as applying to all women," although we have taken care to explain not that they *would* be applied to *all* women but that there was evidence that they already *had been* applied to *large numbers* of women. The technique of putting the most extreme of all possible positions in the mouths of feminists is a common one and not limited to Mack but seems particularly inappropriate in what is supposed to be a scholarly thesis. Mack also claims that the *DSM* classifications have been based not on assumptions about their causes but rather on simple description, although, as described in Chapters 4 and 5 of the present book, that is far from the case for both SDPD and LLPDD.

Another totally false and damaging claim he made, as though it were fact, was that "Caplan also was not happy that she had not been consulted before any decision had been made [about SDPD]." Again, the documentation I had provided to him made it clear that the reasons for my concerns were the lack of scientific basis for their decisions and the process by which they were made.

A further example of his selectivity was his description of the LLPDD committee's literature as showing, in summary, that LLPDD does exist, while failing to report that in the summary the committee had described the research as preliminary and filled with methodological problems. Then, too, he alleges—obviously without checking with many of the advisors—that "most of the advisors" leaned toward classifying PMDD as a mood disorder.

Mack did not appear to notice the holes in the *DSM* group's reasoning, for despite his having claimed that their decisions were based on empirical science, he does not comment on the fact that they also said that the task for *DSM-III* was "to decide if there is an entity clinicians *feel they want to describe* in this way" (p. 79: my italics).

His choice of which information to report is highly selected. For instance, he quotes Sally Severino as it serves his argument but fails to point out that, although she had begun as a staunch advocate of LLPDD, she developed serious reservations about its usefulness and began to speak publicly about that over the years. In another example of his selectivity, he baldly asserts that some form of a premenstrual mental disorder "made ineffective usual treatments for depression," completely failing to consider that, if that were the case, the *DSM* group's pushing of antidepressant drugs would be totally unethical.

Mack seems to share the traditional *DSM* group's views on all the relevant issues in his thesis. For instance, rather than saying that they always believed (or argued) that there was a need for a category like SDPD, his wording was that "there was a continuing *recognition* of the need for such a category" (p. 76: my italics). When noting that Spitzer had added to SDPD the criterion that the label should not be applied if the woman was currently a victim of abuse, he then wrote, "However the feminists were still not pacified." In addition to the bias reflected in his word choice there, he ignored the ample evidence (documented in papers he had apparently read, since they were listed in his bibliography) that such a criterion would not be effective, due to therapists' proven tendency at that time to neglect to ask women about histories of abuse.

p. 134 *Betsy Lehman*   Lehman, 1993, p. 36.

p. 134 *Gail Vines*   Vines, 1993, p. 13.

p. 134 *Marilyn Chase*   Chase, 1993, p. B3.

p. 135 " *'People knew 200 years ago ...'* "   Span, 1993, p. C2.

p. 135 *a memo that Gold had written*   Gold, November 23, 1992.

p. 135 *In another memo*   Gold, March 8, 1993.

p. 136 *they described the existing research*   Gold et al., 1993, p. 75.

p. 136 *Anne Fausto-Sterling's book*   Fausto-Sterling, 1985.

p. 136 *"The trustees of the American ..."*   Span, 1993, p. C2.

p. 137 *What was not widely publicized*   Bernier, 1993.

p. 138 *Not only is it scientifically unwarranted*   Tavris, 1992.

p. 138 *Sally Severino*   Vines, 1993.

p. 138 *As an added twist*   deAngelis, 1993.

p. 139 *Tori deAngelis*   deAngelis, 1993.

p. 139 *In April, a National Public Radio producer*   Ann Goodwin Sides, personal communication, April 1, 1993.

p. 140 *"500,000 is not that many"*   Blamphin, personal communication, March 12, 1993.

p. 140 *His response was*   Frances, personal communication, March 12, 1993.

p. 141 *"The potential occupational ..."*   Gold et al., 1993, p. 74.

p. 141 *In another case* Solomon, 1995.

p. 142 *As a result of a March 12 column*   Landsberg, 1993.

p. 142 *We prepared a paper*   Committee for a Scientific and Responsible *DSM*, 1993.

p. 145 *A woman in her early thirties*   Personal communication, 1992, from a woman who asked not to be identified.

p. 148 *Everyday kinds of harm*   Kendall, 1992; Pirie, 1988; Clare, 1983.

p. 148 *At the very worst*   Kendall, 1992; Mills, 1988.

p. 148 *In a general sense*   Nash, 1994; Gallant and Hamilton, 1988.

p. 148 *Heather Nash*   Nash, 1994.

p. 148 *As Nash wrote*   Nash, 1994, p. 60.

p. 148 *"Despite the fact . . ."*   Nash, 1994, p. 61.

p. 149 *Sheryle Gallant*   Gallant, Popiel, Hoffman, Chakraborty, and Hamilton, 1992.

p. 150 *Indeed, in our book*   Caplan and Caplan, 1994.

p. 150 *we followed in the footsteps*   Fausto-Sterling, 1985; Parlee, 1973, 1978b; Tavris, 1992; Harrison, 1985.

p. 156 *Dr. Dodie Pirie*   Pirie and Smith, 1992, report an "overall reduction [of symptoms] of 42 per cent" from their support groups, in which they help women to understand what is happening to them and to reframe their "negative" feelings (p. 46).

p. 157 *Dendron News*   "Demonstrators bring complaints," 1993.

p. 157 *According to Brooks*   Brooks, personal communication, May 25, 1993.

p. 158 *This technique of trying*   see Kirk and Kutchins, 1992.

p. 158 *"The five female psychiatrists . . ."*   Edmonds, 1993.

p. 158 *Gail Robinson*   Robinson, 1993.

p. 160 *Judith Gold's committee's conclusion*   Gold et al., 1993.

p. 161 *Mary Brown Parlee*   Parlee, 1994.

p. 162 *Then, as we have said*   McFarland, Ross, and DeCourville, 1989.

p. 162 *This hypothesis is borne out*   Pirie and Smith, 1992.

p. 162 *"Doctor, I have terrible PMS"*   Tummon, 1993, personal communication, and Tummon and Kramer, 1994.

p. 163 *For instance, there is a positive correlation*   deAngelis, 1993, p. 32.

p. 163 *Michele Landsberg*   Landsberg, 1993, p. J1.

p. 164 *If women are*   Tavris, 1992.

p. 164 *"If women are depressed . . ."*   deAngelis, 1993, p. 32.

p. 165 *An important and serious*   Cattanach, 1985; *PMS Information and Referral Newsletter*, 1987.

p. 165 *And as Tavris has pointed out*   Tavris, 1993.

p. 166 *"There is . . . no scientific . . ."*   "Menstrual stress cited in child abuse case," 1982.

p. 167 *Irresponsible professionals*   Kendall writes: "Three of the most sensationalist homicide cases were tried in Britain: . . . In all three cases, the charge of murder was reduced to manslaughter because PMS was believed to have diminished the women's responsibility for their actions," but the professionals in the case "kept hidden the violence that these women experienced" (Kendall, 1992, p. 53). Perhaps the lawyers in those cases were not irresponsible but had realistically perceived that a "battered woman's defense" would not be accepted by the court as valid but that a claim of diminished mental capacity in a woman would be more readily accepted.

p. 167 *Dr. Jeffrey Nisker*   Adamick, 1986.

p. 167 *Well into the article*   "Menstrual stress cited in child abuse case," 1982.

Chapter 6

p. 168 *Since becoming aware*   Schwartz, 1993. Schwartz writes: "Consider the findings that a woman who indicates more Antisocial Personality Disorder characteristics than a man is still more likely to be diagnosed as Histrionic, while the inverse is true for a man" (Ford & Widiger, 1989).

p. 169 *We called it Delusional*   Caplan and Eichler, 1989.

p. 169 *Table 1*   Pantony and Caplan, 1991a.

p. 171 *When submitting DDPD*   Caplan and Eichler, 1989.

p. 171 *I did receive a response*   Frances, 1989b.

p. 171 *"I submitted [the DDPD proposal] . . ."*   Caplan, 1989f, p. 1.

p. 172 *I also said*   Ibid., p. 1.

p. 172 *"As we have discussed . . ."*   Frances, 1989c.

p. 173 *the introductory chapter*   APA, 1987.

p. 174 *this information came*   Gunderson, 1989a, p. 2.

p. 174 *a paper they wrote*   Frances et al., 1991.

p. 174 *"constantly tinkering . . ."*   Kutchins and Kirk, in press, Chapter XX, Part IV, p. 17.

p. 175 *"setting a very high threshold . . ."*   Frances, 1989d, p. 1.

p. 175 *Gunderson had written*   Gunderson, 1989c, p. 1.

p. 175 *"Like Allen, I urge you . . ."*   Ibid., p. 1.

p. 175 *"highly unlikely . . ."*   Gunderson, 1989a, p. 1.

p. 176 *"this problem is compounded . . ."*   Ibid.

p. 176 *"the most formidable obstacle . . ."*   Gunderson, 1989b.

p. 176 *On December 5, Frances*   Frances, 1989f.

p. 176 *"A new diagnosis . . ."*   Kutchins and Kirk, in press, Chapter XX, Part IV, p. 20.

p. 177 *"it is folly . . ."*   Frances, 1989a, p. 1.

p. 177 *In the same letter*   Ibid.

p. 177 *"I certainly don't advocate . . ."*   Caplan, 1989a, p. 1.

p. 177 *"there was a rising tone . . ."*   Kutchins and Kirk, in press, Chapter XX, Part IV, p. 21.

p. 178 *On February 26, 1990*   Caplan, 1990b.

p. 178 *on March 5 I wrote*   Caplan, 1990c.

p. 178 *"From my work ..."* Ibid., p. 1.
p. 178 *on March 13, he informed me* Frances, 1990b.
p. 178 *"very much against ..."* Ibid., p. 1.
p. 178 *"would not recommend ..."* Ibid., p. 1.
p. 178 *"literally dozens ..."* Ibid., p. 1.
p. 178 *"They seemed to have had enough ..."* Kutchins and Kirk, in press, Chapter XX, Part IV, p. 22.
p. 178 *our review* published later as Pantony and Caplan, 1991.
p. 180 *"actually appear as part ..."* L. Walker, 1987, p. 183.
p. 180 *The insidiousness of the DSM* Kirk and Kutchins, 1992. This was also pointed out even by Allen Frances's nephew in his undergraduate thesis: Mack, 1994.
p. 181 *a look at its index* American Psychiatric Association, 1987, p. 296.
p. 181 *DSM-IV* American Psychiatric Association, 1994.
p. 182 *The Myth of Women's Masochism* Caplan, 1987.
p. 182 *"How Do They Decide ..."* Caplan, 1991a.
p. 182 *coauthored with no fewer* Frances, Widiger, First, Pincus, Tilly, Miele, and Davis, 1991.
p. 182 *"a careful three-stage ..."* Frances et al., 1991, p. ix.
p. 183 *"widely distributed ..."* Ibid., p. 171.
p. 183 *I am also informed* L. Walker, personal communication, August 1993.
p. 183 *"should come to closure ..."* Frances et al., 1991, p. 171.
p. 183 *"distributed widely ..."* Ibid.
p. 184 *"Response to the DSM Wizard"* Caplan, 1991b.
p. 184 *their handful of colleagues* Pantony and Caplan, 1991.

Chapter 7
p. 185 *George Vaillant* Klerman, Vaillant, Spitzer, and Michels, 1984, p. 544.
p. 185 *Peter Breggin* Breggin, 1991, p. 182.
p. 186 *"DSM-IV is a team effort ..."* APA, 1994a, p. xiii.
p. 187 *"intended to provide ..."* APA, 1994c, p. xx.
p. 187 *Fact Sheet* APA, 1993b, pp. 1–3.
p. 189 *The second sentence* APA, 1994a, p. xv.
p. 189 *"The field trials collected ..."* Ibid., p. xix.
p. 189 *It has been fascinating* Kirk and Kutchins, 1992. This is a claim that Allen Frances's nephew uncritically parrots in his paper: Mack, 1994.
p. 190 *"The major difference ..."* Frances et al., 1991, p. 171.
p. 190 *"On July 1, 1980 ..."* Maxmen, 1985, p. 35.
p. 190 *"Scientific psychiatry ..."* Ibid., p. 31.

p. 190 *Sometimes, it is not* Laidlaw, Malmo, and Associates, 1990; Luborsky, Crits-Cristoph, Mintz, and Auerbach, 1988; Rawlings and Carter, 1977; Umbarger, Morrison, Dalsimer, and Breggin, 1962.

p. 191 *The authors of that first* Kass et al., 1986.

p. 195 *The DSM authors diverge* see Kirk and Kutchins, 1992, for detailed descriptions of these practices.

p. 195 *Another serious problem* Kirk and Kutchins, 1992.

p. 195 *"experimenter bias"* Rosenthal and Jacobson, 1968.

p. 195 *"No full, comprehensive report ..."* Kirk and Kutchins, 1992, p. 127.

p. 196 *This research involved* e.g., Spitzer, Hyler, and Williams, 1980; Williams, 1985.

p. 197 *Kirk and Kutchins have traced* Kirk and Kutchins, 1992.

p. 198 *three publications* Spitzer, Forman, and Nee, 1979; APA, 1980; Hyler, Williams, and Spitzer, 1982.

p. 198 *Spitzer, Forman, and Nee* Spitzer, Forman, and Nee, 1979.

p. 198 *"reliability is quite good"* Ibid., p. 820.

p. 200 *In a second study* Hyler, Williams, and Spitzer, 1982.

p. 200 *In the* DSM-III *itself* APA, 1980.

p. 201 *Kirk and Kutchins describe* Kirk and Kutchins, 1992.

p. 201 *"quite good, and in general ..."* Spitzer, Williams, and Skodol, 1980, p. 154.

p. 201 *"The field trials themselves ..."* Kirk and Kutchins, 1992, pp. 157, 179.

p. 202 *"the highest-ranking psychiatrist ..."* Kirk and Kutchins, 1992, p. 6.

p. 202 *"science in the service of healing ..."* Klerman et al., 1984, p. 541.

p. 202 *However, an investigation* Cantwell, Russell, Mattison, and Will, 1979.

p. 202 *When it came time* Kirk and Kutchins, 1992.

p. 202 *Some of their work apparently* Kirk and Kutchins, 1992.

p. 202 *Whereas the field trials* APA, 1987.

p. 203 *Although no reliability* Williams, Gibbon, First, Spitzer, Davies, Borus, Howes, Kane, Pope, Rounsaville, and Wittchen, 1992.

p. 203 *The analogy used* Mirowsky and Ross, 1989.

p. 204 *"exhaustively researched"* APA, August 1993, p. 1.

p. 204 *"by groups of symptoms ..."* Ibid., p. 1.

p. 204 *"The process of systematically ..."* APA, August 1993, p. 3.

p. 205 *"open process"* APA, August 1993, p. 4.

p. 205 *According to Lenore Walker* cited by Armstrong, 1993, p.

155. Also, Kutchins and Kirk (in press) say that, "For Spitzer and his committees, creating a new diagnostic category was something of a house specialty; they had done it numerous times before. The recipe was easy: pick a label, provide a general description based on clinical wisdom, develop a menu of 'diagnostic criteria,' check the proposed criteria with advocates for the new category, decide how many criteria had to be met to use the diagnosis, counter opposition if any, and, presto!, you had a new mental disorder ready to serve" (Kutchins and Kirk, in press, Chapter XX, Part II, pp. 1–2).

p. 205 *Remember that the APA*   Caplan, 1987.
p. 206 *"to obtain data . . ."*   Letter from Work Group, 1986.
p. 207 *"The questionnaire . . . asks . . ."*   Braude, 1986.
p. 207 *Kutchins and Kirk report*   Kutchins and Kirk, in press, Chapter XX, Part II, p. 34.
p. 207 *Even so, this piece*   Kutchins and Kirk, in press.
p. 208 *Wendy Schwartz*   Schwartz, 1993.
p. 208 *Judith Herman*   Herman, 1988.
p. 208 *Gans and myself*   Caplan and Gans, 1991.
p. 208 *"like adding together slightly rotten . . ."*   Caplan, 1989, letter to Fiester, November 28.
p. 208 *The Personality Disorders*   American Psychiatric Association's DSM-IV Personality Disorders Work Group, 1991.
p. 209 *Allen Frances's statement*   Frances, 1989b, p. 1.
p. 209 *In regard to LLPDD*   Fausto-Sterling, 1985; Caplan, McCurdy-Myers, and Gans, 1992a; Tavris, 1992.
p. 209 *This last move*   Gold et al., 1993.
p. 210 *"As is the case . . ."*   Ibid., p. 12.
p. 210 *"The criteria as proposed . . ."*   Ibid., p. 16.
p. 211 *"The distinction between affective . . ."*   Ibid., p. 64.
p. 211 *"There are still only . . ."*   Ibid., p. 66.
p. 211 *the more a woman believes*   McFarland, Ross, and DeCourville, 1989.
p. 211 *emotions reported retrospectively*   Parlee, 1982.
p. 211 *Just knowing that one*   Hamilton and Gallant, 1993.
p. 211 *When women are asked*   Ibid. and McFarlane, Martin, and Williams, 1988; Parlee, 1982.
p. 211 *Similarly, when women*   Ruble, 1977; Klebanov and Jemmott, 1992; Sommer, 1973.
p. 211 *Indeed, even in women*   Hamilton and Gallant, 1993.
p. 211 *In fact, women who report*   Hamilton, Alagna, and Sharpe, 1985; Gallant and Hamilton, 1988; Fradkin and Firestone, 1986.

p. 212 *When researchers compared* McFarlane, Martin, and Williams, 1988.

p. 212 *Finally, women who have* Gallant, Popiel, and Hoffman, in press.

p. 212 *Kaye Lee Pantony and I* Pantony and Caplan, 1993.

p. 215 *Under the category of "Encopresis"* APA, 1994a, pp. 63–65.

p. 217 *In one fell swoop* Caplan, 1994a.

p. 218 *June Larkin and I* Larkin and Caplan, 1992.

p. 219 *"new diagnoses . . ."* APA, 1991b, p. A-6.

p. 220 *"How Do They Decide Who Is Normal?"* Caplan, 1991a.

p. 220 *Frances and his colleagues* Frances et al., 1991, p. 173.

p. 220 *"controversies that detract . . ."* Ibid.

p. 220 *"quiet consideration . . ."* Ibid.

p. 220 *In their Personality Disorders* APA, 1991a.

p. 221 *Arthur Nikelly* Nikelly, 1992.

p. 221 *"Psychiatry and Society"* Tsuang, Tohen, and Murphy, 1988, p. 764.

p. 221 *"I read the [DSM-III-R] compiler's . . ."* Dumont, 1987, p. 9

p. 222 *Table 1* Larkin and Caplan, 1992, pp. 20–22.

Chapter 8

p. 227 *You're Smarter Than They Make You Feel* Caplan, 1994b.

p. 227 *As I have said* Caplan, 1994b.

p. 228 *Most people find* Kovel (1988) has written: "The age-old dream of science, that of total control by man over nature, embodied here in the endless proliferation of categories, lists and 'decision-trees,' becomes thereby an instrument of domination" (p. 135).

p. 228 *At best, then* Viscott, 1972.

p. 230 *Furthermore, the more diagnostic* Rothblum, Solomon, and Albee, 1986.

p. 231 *"because it increases . . ."* APA, 1994b, p. 9.

p. 231 *Furthermore, mental health researchers* Rothblum, Solomon, and Albee, 1986, p. 167.

p. 231 *The only kind of "treatment"* see Gold et al., 1993, as well as Judith Gold's remarks on many of the radio and television shows and in many of the print media articles mentioned in Chapter 9.

p. 231 *"stand to make a great deal of money . . ."* Tavris, 1992, p. 141, quoting Parlee, 1989. And Brown and Cooksey, 1993, note "the necessity of using DSM criteria for patients in clinical trials by European pharmaceutical companies if they want their wares to be accepted by the U.S. Food and

Drug Administration" (p. 12).

p. 232 *"too big a market . . ."*   Tavris, 1992, p. 158.

p. 232 *At a recent meeting*   Psychologists' Society of Saskatchewan, 1994.

p. 232 *"Appendix D in DSM-III-R . . ."*   Zimmerman, 1988, pp. 1135–37.

p. 233 *"The drug companies provide . . ."*   Breggin, 1991, p. 345.

p. 233 *"The psychiatric newspapers . . ."*   Ibid., p. 345.

p. 233 *The drug companies also*   Ibid., p. 345.

p. 234 *"Marxist" and "paranoid"*   Ibid., p. 352.

p. 234 *Fred Gottlieb*   Gottlieb, Oct. 1984, p. 1333.

p. 234 *"It is the task of APA . . ."*   Fink, 1986, p. 16.

p. 234 *"organized psychiatry is big business . . ."*   Breggin, 1991, pp. 366–67.

p. 235 *Insurance companies*   Armstrong, 1993; Sharkey, 1994.

p. 235 *As a result, therapists*   Brown and Cooksey, 1993.

p. 235 *the gamut of dangers*   Armstrong, 1993; Breggin, 1991; Burstow and Weitz, 1988; Chamberlin, 1978; Finkler, 1993; Girard and Collett, 1983; Greene, 1992; Kaminer, 1992; Kitzinger, 1990; Millett, 1991; Mithers, 1994; Nelkin and Tancredi, 1989; Scheff, 1966; Walker, 1993.

p. 235 *psychiatry as a profession*   As Louise Armstrong (1993) writes: "Indeed, on diagnosis depends psychiatry's authority, its assertion that it is in fact a medical specialty, a science. The naming of the diseases (disorders) stakes the claim of expertise, and the right of intervention" (p. 131).

p. 235 *"won cultural jurisdiction . . ."*   Kirk and Kutchins, 1992, p. 10.

p. 235 *Joseph English*   English, 1993, pp. 1294–95.

p. 236 *"at the bottom of the totem pole . . ."*   Kirk and Kutchins, 1992, p. 10.

p. 236 *"solidif[y] the claim . . ."*   Brown and Cooksey, 1993, p. 6.

p. 236 *Canadian Mental Health Association's*   Canadian Mental Health Association's Women and Mental Health Committee, 1987.

p. 237 *Both categories make it easier*   Caplan, 1989.

p. 237 *Carol Tavris*   Carol Tavris, 1992, has written: ". . . the idea that menstruation is a debilitating condition that makes women unfit for work has its own cycle. It comes and goes in phase with women's participation in the labor market . . . research findings about menstruation change over time, corresponding to women's role in the work force. At the start of World War II, for example, studies suddenly found that menstruation and 'premenstrual tension' were not problems for working women. One researcher, who wrote in 1934 that menstruation was debilitating, changed her mind after the war began ... [but after WWII, the news changed again] ... research on PMS erupted in the 1970s, a decade when, as Martin observes, 'women had made greater incursions into the paid work force for the first time without the aid of a major war.' [Martin, 1987, p. 120] ... Mary Brown Parlee ... observes that psychologists who were studying menstruation tended to focus on normal menstrual cycles. The big money, the big grants, increasingly went to the biomedical researchers, on the assumption that PMS was a disease ... [Parlee, 1989]"(Tavris, 1992, pp. 139–41).

p. 237 *Louise Armstrong* Armstrong, 1993, 1994.

Chapter 9
p. 242 *Furthermore, as I have written elsewhere* Caplan, 1994b.
p. 242 *Although it is true* Caplan and Gans, 1991.
p. 245 *Jean Hamilton* Hamilton, 1987/88.
p. 245 *"tainted motives ..."* Ibid., p. 9.
p. 246 *"Nonetheless, an exact ..."* Ibid., p. 9.
p. 246 *"Instead of using a neutral ..."* Ibid., pp. 9–10.
p. 253 *"the standards for proposed ..."* Goode, 1993, p. 50.
p. 253 *"a serious exploration ..."* Seligmann and Gelman, 1993, p. 66.
p. 253 *"the new definition ..."* Socha, 1993, p. F8.
p. 253 *Tori deAngelis* deAngelis, 1993.
p. 254 *"a task force ..."* Seligmann and Gelman, 1993, p. 66.
p. 254 *deAngelis's use* deAngelis, 1993, p. 32.
p. 254 *"Caplan contends"* Ness, 1993, p. A16.
p. 254 *Miles Socha* Socha, 1993.
p. 254 *Marilyn Linton* Linton, 1993, p. 52.
p. 255 *"threatening to sue"* Lehman, 1993, p. 36.
p. 255 *"not-even-slightly-veiled threat ..."* Span, 1993, p. C2.
p. 255 *a published paper* Caplan, 1991a.
p. 255 *"[Caplan's letter to the APA] ..."* Clarification, 1993, p. A2.
p. 256 *Lindsay Scotton* Scotton, 1993.
p. 256 *"By saying that ..."* Lehman, 1993, p. A1.
p. 256 *"misleading" title* Span, 1993, p. C2.
p. 257 *"So far, fears ..."* Ibid.
p. 257 *a top APA administrator's* Cornacchia, 1993.

p. 257 *that we were "outraged"* Seligmann and Gelman, 1993.

p. 257 *"threatening to sue"* Lehman, 1993, p. 36.

p. 258 *Reporters ignored* e.g., deAngelis, 1993; Span, 1993.

p. 258 *compelling evidence* Gallant, Popiel, Hoffman, Chakraborty, and Hamilton, 1992.

p. 258 *"remains to be shown"* Span, 1993, p. C2.

p. 258 *Carol Ness* Ness, 1993.

p. 259 *"according to standard practice"* Solomon, 1993, p. 33.

p. 259 *Chase's otherwise good article* Chase, 1993.

p. 260 *Related to this* Ness, 1993; Feminists assail, 1993; Span, 1993; Vines, 1993.

p. 260 *Carol Tavris* Tavris, 1993.

p. 260 *Michele Landsberg* Landsberg, 1993.

p. 260 *Kristina Stockwood* Stockwood, 1993.

p. 260 *Gail Vines* Vines, 1993

p. 261 *"The comparable excuse . . ."* Tavris, 1993, p. B7.

p. 261 *"just a couple of decades ago . . ."* Landsberg, 1993, p. J1.

p. 262 *"the psychiatric profession . . ."* Solomon, 1993, pp. 32–33.

p. 262 *"Dr. Caplan and her associates . . ."* Donaldson and King-well, 1993, p. A23.

Chapter 10

p. 273 *As a result* Kinsbourne and Caplan, 1979.

p. 275 *As Phil Brown* Brown and Cooksey, 1993, p. 3.

p. 275 *Maureen Graham* Graham, 1994.

p. 275 *Nayyar Javed* Javed, 1994.

p. 276 *It is especially tragic* Martinez, 1994, p. B01

p. 277 *"In the turbulent 1960s . . ."* Brown, 1990, p. 388.

p. 278 *"Up to 75 percent . . ."* Sleek, 1994, p. 28.

p. 278 *so much loneliness Albee* writes about "a society composed largely of lonely persons" whose loneliness leads them to seek therapy, where they are labeled mentally ill: Albee, 1990, p. 378.

p. 279 *as Albee observes* Albee, 1990, p. 382. Albee also writes: "Only with radical social changes leading to a just society will there be a reduction in the incidence of emotional problems." (p. 377).

p. 279 *Louise Armstrong* Armstrong, 1993, writes: ". . . exhausted by the apparent futility of efforts at social change, the public was more susceptible to the psy sector's salesmanship of personal 'mental health' solutions for socially related distress. The greater the sense of helplessness in the face of oppression—in the face of real events—the greater the appeal of the distractions offered by psy-think" (p. 156). In a related vein, Castel, Castel, and Lovell, 1982, note ". . . the persistent pattern of American welfare policy, denying that poverty is a social and political problem, instead approaching welfare recipients as cases for psychological and moral examination" (p. 9). Similar reasoning applies to the targets of racism, sexism, ageism, classism, homophobia, prejudice against people with disabilities, and so on. And Scheff says: ". . . mental illness may be more usefully considered to be a social status than a disease, since the symptoms of mental illness are vaguely defined and widely distributed, and the definition of behavior as symptomatic of mental illness is usually dependent upon social rather than medical contingencies" (1966, pp. 128–29).

p. 280 *"Native people who drink . . ."*   Finkler, 1993, p. 73.
p. 281 *David Randall*   Randall, 1994.
p. 282 *"Many people and facilities . . ."*   Brown and Cooksey, 1993, p. 3.
p. 282 *George Albee*   Albee, 1990, p. 381.
p. 284 *When alternative*   Caplan, 1993.
p. 285 *Judi Chamberlin*   Chamberlin, 1978, p. 8.
p. 285 *Psychoanalyst Evelyne Schwaber*   Schwaber, 1983.
p. 286 *Joel Kovel*   Kovel, 1988.
p. 287 *"secured into a system . . ."*   Kovel, 1988, p. 134.
p. 287 *"the person and his/her . . ."*   Kovel, 1988, p. 145.
p. 287 *In one APA publication*   August 1993, p. 1.
p. 288 *"abide by their codes . . ."*   Kirk and Kutchins, 1992, p. 243.
p. 289 *But it has been said*   Antony, 1993.

Bibliography

*Bibliography items that are marked with an asterisk (*) are published materials that, to varying degrees, include questioning, critical-thinking perspectives on either the *DSM* itself or issues addressed in this book.

†Bibliography items that are marked with a dagger (†) are the subjects of Chapter 9, on the media.

*Adamick, Paula. 1986. Pre-menstrual syndrome cited in defence of stabbing. *Toronto Star*. December 11, p. A19.

Advertisement. 1986. Blurb by Donald Godwin, Chairman and Professor of Psychiatry in the Department of Psychiatry at the University of Kansas, regarding *Contemporary directions in psychopathology: Toward the DSM-IV*, edited by Theodore Millon and Gerald Klerman. Behavioral Science Book Service. November.

*Albee, George. 1990. The futility of psychotherapy. *Journal of Mind and Behavior* 11, 369–84.

American Psychiatric Association. 1994a. *Diagnostic and statistical manual of mental disorders-IV*. Washington, D.C.: American Psychiatric Association.

American Psychiatric Association. 1994b. *DSM-IV update*. Washington, D.C.: American Psychiatric Association. March.

American Psychiatric Association. 1994c. *DSM-IV sourcebook*. Washington, D.C.: American Psychiatric Association.

American Psychiatric Association. 1993a. *DSM-IV update*. Washington, D.C.: American Psychiatric Association. January/February.

American Psychiatric Association. 1993b. *Fact sheet: Psychiatric diagnosis and the diagnostic and statistical manual of mental disorders (fourth edition), DSM-IV*. Washington, D.C.: American Psychiatric Association. August.

American Psychiatric Association's *DSM-IV* Work Group on Personality Disorders. 1991a. Minutes for September 19–21.

American Psychiatric Association. 1991b. *DSM-IV options*. September 1.

American Psychiatric Association. 1987. *Diagnostic and statistical manual of mental disorders–III–R*. Washington, D.C.: American Psychiatric Association.

American Psychiatric Association. 1980. *Diagnostic and statistical manual of mental disorders–III*. Washington, D.C.: American Psychiatric Association.

*Antony, Louise. 1993. Quine as feminist: The radical import of naturalized epistemology. In Louise Antony and Charlotte Witt (Eds.), *A mind of one's own: Feminist essays on reason and objectivity.* Boulder, Colo.: Westview, pp. 185–225.

*Armstrong, Louise. 1994. *Rocking the cradle of sexual politics: What happened when women said incest.* Reading, Mass.: Addison-Wesley.

*Armstrong, Louise. 1993. *And they call it help: The psychiatric policing of America's children.* Reading, Mass.: Addison-Wesley.

*Bayer, R. 1981. *Homosexuality and American psychiatry: The politics of diagnosis.* New York: Basic Books.

*Bentall, Richard. 1992. A proposal to classify happiness as a psychiatric disorder. *Journal of Medical Ethics* 18:94–98.

Berger, G. 1984. *PMS: Premenstrual syndrome.* Claremont, Calif.: Hunterhouse.

Bernier, George M. 1993. Letter. February 2.

Bishop, Joan E. H. 1989. Personal communication. December 12.

Blamphin, John. 1993. Personal communication. March 12.

*Braude, Marjorie. 1986. Concerns about APA questionnaire on personality disorders. *American Journal of Psychiatry*, 143, 1309.

*Breggin, Peter R. 1991. *Toxic psychiatry: Why therapy, empathy, and love must replace the drugs, electroshock, and biochemical theories of the "new psychiatry."* New York: St. Martin's Press.

*Broverman, Inge, Donald Broverman, Frank Clarkson, Paul Rosenkrantz, and Susan Vogel. 1970. Sex-role stereotypes and clinical judgments of mental health. *Journal of Consulting and Clinical Psychology* 34:1–7.

*Brown, Laura. 1986. Report from the latest meetings on the DSM-III-R. *Feminist Therapists' Institute Interchange.* July 3.

*Brown, Phil. 1990. The name game: Toward a sociology of diagnosis. *The Journal of Mind and Behavior* 11:385–406.

*Brown, Phil. 1987. Diagnostic conflict and contradiction in psychiatry. *Journal of Health and Social Behavior* 28:37–50.

*Brown, Phil, and Elizabeth Cooksey. 1993. Spinning on its axes: DSM and the social construction of psychiatric diagnosis. Unpublished paper.

*Burstow, Bonnie, and Don Weitz, eds. 1988. *Shrink resistant: The struggle against psychiatry in Canada.* Vancouver, B.C.: New Star Books.

*Butler, Robert N. 1975. *Why survive? Being old in America.* New York: Harper and Row.

*Canadian Mental Health Association's Women and Mental

Health Committee. 1987. *Women and mental health in Canada: Strategies for change.* Toronto: CMHA.

*Cantwell, Dennis, A. Russell, R. Mattison, and L. Will. 1979. A comparison of DSM-II and DSM-III in the diagnosis of childhood psychiatric disorders. *Archives of General Psychiatry 36,* 1208–22.

*Caplan, Paula J. 1994a. *The myth of women's masochism.* Toronto: University of Toronto Press.

*Caplan, Paula J. 1994b. *You're smarter than they make you feel: How the experts intimidate us and what we can do about it.* New York: Free Press.

*Caplan, Paula J. 1993. The justice system's endorsement of mental health assessors' sexism and other forms of bias. In B. Dickens and M. Ouellette (Eds.), *Health care, ethics and law/Soins de santé, ethique, et droit.* canadian Institute for the Administration of Justice/Institut canadien d'administration de la justice. Les editions Themis, pp. 79–87.

*Caplan, Paula J. 1992. Driving us crazy: How oppression damages women's mental health and what we can do about it. *Women and Therapy* 12:5–28.

*Caplan, Paula J. 1991a. How *do* they decide who is normal? The bizarre, but true, tale of the *DSM* process. *Canadian Psychology/Psychologie Canadienne* 32:162–70.

Caplan, Paula J. 1991b. Response to the DSM wizard. *Canadian Psychology/Psychologie Canadienne* 32, 174–75.

Caplan, Paula J. 1990a. Letter to Allen Frances. November 8.

Caplan, Paula J. 1990b. Letter to Allen Frances. February 26.

Caplan, Paula J. 1990c. Letter to Susan Fiester. March 5.

*Caplan, Paula J. 1989a. *Don't blame mother: Mending the mother-daughter relationship.* New York: Harper and Row.

Caplan, Paula J. 1989b. Comments on Susan Fiester's "Self-defeating Personality Disorder: A Review of Data and Recommendations for *DSM-IV*." Unpublished paper. November 28.

Caplan, Paula J. 1989c. Letter to Allen Frances. November 8.

Caplan, Paula J. 1989d. Letter to John Gunderson. November 8.

Caplan, Paula J. 1989e. Letter to Susan Fiester. November 28.

Caplan, Paula J. 1989f. Letter to John Gunderson. June 23.

Caplan, Paula J. 1989g. Letter to Susan Fiester. May.

*Caplan, Paula J. 1987. *The myth of women's masochism.* New York: Signet. Includes new chapter on SDPD called "Afterword: A warning."

Caplan, Paula J. 1986. Letter to APA Board Members. December 5.

*Caplan, Paula J. 1985. *The myth of women's masochism.* New York: E.P. Dutton (original hardcover edition).

*Caplan, Paula J. 1984. The myth of women's masochism. *American Psychologist* 39:130–39.

*Caplan, Paula J. 1981. *Between women: Lowering the barriers.* Toronto: Personal Library.

*Caplan, Paula J., and Jeremy B. Caplan. 1994. *Thinking critically about research on sex and gender.* New York: HarperCollins.

Caplan, Paula J., and Margrit Eichler. 1989. A proposal for Delusional Dominating Personality Disorder. Unpublished paper.

*Caplan, Paula J., and Maureen Gans. 1991. Is there empirical justification for the category of "Self-defeating Personality Disorder"? *Feminism and Psychology* 1:263–78.

*Caplan, Paula J., and Ian Hall-McCorquodale. 1985a. Mother-blaming in major clinical journals. *American Journal of Orthopsychiatry* 55:345–53.

*Caplan, Paula J., and Ian Hall-McCorquodale. 1985b. The scapegoating of mothers: A call for change. *American Journal of Orthopsychiatry* 55:610–13.

*Caplan, Paula J., Joan McCurdy-Myers, and Maureen Gans. 1992a. Should "premenstrual syndrome" be called a psychiatric abnormality? *Feminism and Psychology* 2:27–44.

*Caplan, Paula J., Joan McCurdy-Myers, and Maureen Gans. 1992b. Reply to Mary Brown Parlee's commentary on PMS and psychiatric abnormality. *Feminism and Psychology* 2:109.

*Capponi, Pat. 1992. *Upstairs in the crazy house: The life of a psychiatric survivor.* Toronto: Viking.

Carmen, Elaine (Hilberman). 1985. Masochistic personality disorder DSM-III-R: Critique. November 7. Unpublished.

*Carniol, Ben. 1987. *Case critical: Challenging social work in Canada.* Toronto: Between the Lines.

Carson, Robert C. 1994. Continuity in personality and its derangements. Presented in Session No. 4180, American Psychological Association convention. Los Angeles. August 15.

*Castel, Robert, Francoise Castel, and Anne Lovell. 1982. *The psychiatric society.* New York: Columbia University Press.

*Cattanach, J. 1985. Estrogen deficiency after tubal ligation. *Lancet* (April): 847–49.

*Chamberlin, Judi. 1994. A psychiatric survivor speaks out. *Feminism and Psychology* 4:284–87.

*Chamberlin, Judi. 1978. *On our own: Patient-controlled alternatives to the mental health system.* New York: Hawthorn.

*Chapman, S. 1979. Advertising and psychotropic drugs: The place of myth in ideological reproduction. *Social Science and Medicine* 13A:751–64.

†Chase, Marilyn. 1993. Version of PMS called disorder by psychiatrists. *Wall Street Journal*, May 28, B1, B3.

*Chesler, Phyllis. 1972. *Women and madness.* Garden City, N.Y.: Doubleday.

*Chrisler, Joan, and Joan Howard, eds. 1992. *New directions in feminist psychology.* New York: Springer.

*Chrisler, Joan, and K. B. Levy. 1990. The media construct a menstrual monster: A content analysis of PMS articles in the popular press. *Women and Health* 16:89–104.

*Clare, A. 1983. The relationship between psychopathology and the menstrual cycle. In Sharon Golub, ed., *Lifting the curse of menstruation.* New York: Haworth.

†Clarification. 1993. *Washington Post.* July 16, p. A2.

*Cohen, David, ed. 1990. Special issue: Challenging the therapeutic state: Critical perspectives on psychiatry and the mental health system. *The Journal of Mind and Behavior* 11, nos. 3, 4 (summer/autumn).

*Cole, Carolyn, and Elaine E. Barney. 1987. Safeguards and the therapeutic window: A group treatment strategy for adult incest survivors. *American Journal of Orthopsychiatry,* 57, 601–9.

Committee for a Scientific and Responsible DSM. 1993. Before you vote on the DSM-IV proposal about Premenstrual Syndrome, please read this. Position paper sent to American Psychiatric Association's Legislative Assembly and Executive.

Committee on Women, American Psychiatric Association. 1985. Issues in the acceptance of masochistic personality disorder. Autumn. Unpublished.

*Conrad, P. 1980. On the medicalization of deviance and social control. In D. Ingleby, ed., *Critical psychiatry.* New York: Pantheon.

Corlett, Dianne. 1993. Letter to Allen Frances, August 11.

†Cornacchia, Cheryl. 1993. Is PMS a mental illness? *The Gazette,* August 2, pp. A1, F2.

*Coughlin, P. C. 1990. Premenstrual syndrome: How marital satisfaction and role choice affect symptom severity. *Social Work* 35:351–55.

*Dabbs, James M., Jr., and Robin Morris. 1990. Testosterone, social class, and antisocial behavior in a sample of 4,462 men. *Psychological Science* 1:209–11.

†deAngelis, Tori. 1993. Controversial diagnosis is voted into lat-

est DSM: Opponents cite potential of harm to women. *American Psychological Association Monitor*, September, pp. 32–33.

*de Girolamo, Giovanni. In press. WHO studies on schizophrenia: An overview of the results and their implications for the understanding of the disorder. In Peter Breggin and H. Mark Stern, eds., *Psychotherapy and the psychotic patient*. New York: Haworth. Also a double issue of the journal *The Psychotherapy Patient*.

*DeHardt, Doris. 1992. Feminist therapy with heterosexual couples: The ultimate issue is domination. *Feminism and Psychology* 2:498–501.

*Demonstrators bring complaints to APA's 1993 annual meeting. 1993. *Psychiatric News*. June 18.

*Dendron. 1993. Special issue on APA and *DSM-IV*. P.O. Box 11284, Eugene, OR 97440-3484.

*Denmark, Florence, Nancy Felipe Russo, Irene Hanson Frieze, and Jeri A.Sechzer. 1988. Guidelines for avoiding sexism in psychological research. *American Psychologist* 43:582–85.

*dePaul, A. 1986. Defining new diseases of the mind. Feminist groups complain that a diagnosis of PMS will cause discrimination. *Washington Post Health*, March 5.

*deSousa, Ronald. 1972. II. The politics of mental illness. *Inquiry* 15:187–202.

†Donaldson, Gail, and Mark Kingwell. 1993. Who gets to decide who's normal? *The Globe and Mail*, May 18, p. A23.

*Dumont, Matthew. 1994. Deep in the heart of Chelsea. *Mother Jones*, March/April, pp. 60-64.

*Dumont, Matthew. 1987. A diagnostic parable (First edition–unrevised). *READINGS: A Journal of Reviews and Commentary in Mental Health*. December, 9–12.

Edmonds, Sara. 1993. Personal communication. May 24.

*Ehrenreich, Barbara, and Deirdre English. 1973. *Witches, midwives and nurses: A history of women healers*. Old Westbury: The Feminist Press.

English, Joseph. 1993. Presidential address: Patient care for the twenty-first century: Asserting professional values within economic restraints. *American Journal of Psychiatry* 150:1293–97.

*Faludi, Susan. 1991. *Backlash: The undeclared war against women*. New York: Crown, p. 356.

Fauman, Michael. 1994. *Study guide to DSM-IV*. Washington, D.C.: American Psychiatric Association.

*Fausto-Sterling, Anne. 1985. *Myths of gender: Biological theories about men and women*. New York: Basic Books.

†**Feminists assail move to call PMS a disorder.** 1993. *News and Leader*, May 30, p. 10A.

Fiester, Susan. 1989a. Letter to Paula Caplan. July 10.

Fiester, Susan. 1989b. Letter to Paula Caplan. November 17.

*****Findley, Timothy.** 1993. *Headhunter.* Toronto: Harper-Collins.

Fink, P. J. 1987. Foreword. In B. E. Ginsburg and B. F. Carter, eds., *Premenstrual syndrome.* New York: Plenum.

Fink, Paul. 1986. Position statement. *Psychiatric News*, December 19, p. 16.

*****Finkler, Lilith.** 1993. Notes for feminist therapists on the lives of psychiatrized women. *Canadian Woman Studies* 13:72–74.

*****Fisher, B., P. Giblin, and M. Hoopes.** 1982. Healthy family functioning: What therapists say and what families want. *Journal of Marital and Family Therapy* 8:273–84.

*****Ford, M.R., and T.A. Widiger.** 1989. Sex bias in the diagnosis of histrionic and antisocial personality disorders. *Journal of Consulting and Clinical Psychology* 57, 301–5.

*****Fradkin, B., and P. Firestone.** 1986. Premenstrual tension, expectancy, and mother-child relations. *Journal of Behavioral medicine* 9:245–59.

Frances, Allen. 1993. Personal communication. March 12.

Frances, Allen. 1990a. Letter to Paula Caplan. February 7.

Frances, Allen. 1990b. Letter to Allen Frances. March 13.

Frances, Allen. 1989a. Letter to Paula Caplan. October 26.

Frances, Allen. 1989b. Letter to Paula Caplan. June 12.

Frances, Allen. 1989c. Letter to Paula Caplan. July 24.

Frances, Allen. 1989d. Letter to Doris Howard. August 15.

Frances, Allen. 1989e. Letter to Paula Caplan. October 16.

Frances, Allen. 1989f. Letter to Paula Caplan. December 5.

Frances, Allen. 1988. Memorandum to DSM-IV Work Group. September 19.

Frances, Allen, Thomas A. Widiger, Michael B. First, Harold A. Pincus, Sarah M. Tilly, Gloria M. Miele, and Wendy W. Davis. 1991. *DSM-IV*: Toward a more empirical diagnostic system. *Canadian Psychology/Psychologie Canadienne* 32:171–73.

*****Frank, Jerome.** 1949. *Courts on trial: Myth and reality in American justice.* Princeton, N.J.: Princeton University Press.

*****Gabel, Peter.** 1984. The phenomenology of rights-consciousness and the pact of the withdrawn selves. *Texas Law Review* 62:1563–99.

*****Gallant, Sheryle (Allagna), and Jean A. Hamilton.** 1988. On a premenstrual psychiatric diagnosis: What's in a name? *Professional Psychology: Research and Practice* 19:271–78.

*Gallant, Sheryle, D. A. Popiel, and D. H. Hoffman. In press. The role of psychological variables in the experience of premenstrual symptoms. *Proceedings of the Society for Menstrual Cycle Research.*

*Gallant, Sheryle, Debra Popiel, Denise Hoffman, Prabir Chakraborty, and Jean Hamilton. 1992. Using daily ratings to confirm Premenstrual Syndrome/Late Luteal Phase Dysphoric Disorder. Part II. What makes a "real" difference? *Psychosomatic Medicine* 54:167–81.

*Gartrell, Nanette, ed. 1994. Bringing ethics alive: Feminist ethics in psychotherapy practice. *Women and Therapy* 15 (special issue).

*Gilligan, Carol. 1982. *In a different voice: Psychological theory and women's development.* Cambridge: Harvard University Press.

*Girard, Judy, and Cathy Collett. 1983. Dykes and psychs. *Resources for Feminist Research/Documentation sur la Recherche Feministe XII*, 47–50.

*Goffman, Erving. 1961. *Asylums: Essays on the social situation of mental patients and other inmates.* Garden City, N.Y.: Anchor.

Gold, Judith, J. Endicott, B. Parry, S. Severino, N. Stotland, and E. Frank. 1993. DSM-IV literature review: Late luteal phase dysphoric disorder. Unpublished paper, distributed by American Psychiatric Association.

*Goleman, Daniel. 1990. New paths to mental health put strains on some healers. *The New York Times*, May 17, p. A2.

†Goode, Erica E. 1992. Sick, or just quirky? *U.S. News and World Report*, February 10, pp. 49–50.

*Gotkin, Janet, and Paul Gotkin. 1975. *Too much anger, too many tears: A personal triumph over psychiatry.* New York: Quadrangle.

*Gottlieb, Fred. 1984. Report. *American Journal of Psychiatry*, p. 1333.

Graham, Maureen. 1994. Panel presentation about *DSM*. Psychologists' Society of Saskatchewan conference. Regina, Sask., Canada. April 28.

*Greenberg, Irwin M. 1980. Social Calvinism, free will, etiology, and treatment. In John Talbott, ed., *State mental hospitals: Problems and potentials.* New York: Human Sciences Press, pp. 33–46.

*Greenberg, R. P., and S. Fisher. 1989. Examining antidepressant effectiveness: Findings, ambiguities, and some vexing puzzles. In S. Fisher and R. P. Greenberg, eds., *The limits of biological treatments for psychological distress: Comparisons with psychotherapy and placebo.* Hillsdale, N.J.: Lawrence Erlbaum, pp. 1–37.

*Greene, Beverly. 1992. Still here: A perspective on psychother-
apy with African American women. In Joan Chrisler and Doris
Howard, eds., *New directions in feminist psychology.* New York:
Springer, pp. 13–25.

†Grimes, Charlotte. 1993. Psychiatrists are crazy, man. *St. Louis
Post-Dispatch,* July 15.

*Guidelines for providers of psychological services to ethnic,
linguistic, and culturally diverse populations. 1993. *American
Psychologist* 48:45–48.

Gunderson, John. 1989a. Letter to Paula Caplan. October 16.

Gunderson, John. 1989b. Letter to Paula Caplan. November 14.

Gunderson, John. 1989c. Letter to Paula Caplan. August 23.

*Hamilton, Jean. 1987/88. Is media coverage on the diagnostic
controversy an index of history-in-the-making for women in science? *Newsletter of the National Coalition for Women's Mental
Health,* Fall 1987/Spring 1988, pp. 9–11.

*Hamilton, Jean A., Sheryle Alagna, and K. Sharpe. 1985. Cog-
nitive approaches to understanding and treating premenstrual
depression. In O. J. Osofsky and S. J. Blumenthal, eds., *Premenstrual syndrome: Current findings and future directions.* Washington, D.C.: American Psychiatric Press, pp. 66–83.

*Hamilton, Jean, Sheryle Alagna, Barbara Parry, Elizabeth
Herz, Susan Blumenthal, and Cynthia Conrad. 1985. An
update on premenstrual depressions: Evaluation and treatment. In Judith Gold, ed., *The psychiatric implications of menstruation.* Washington, D.C.: American Psychiatric
Association, pp. 3–19.

*Hamilton, Jean A., and Sheryle Gallant. 1993. Premenstrual
syndromes: A health psychology critique of biomedically-
oriented research. In R. J. Gatchel and E. B. Blanchard, eds.,
Psychophysiological disorders. Washington, D.C.: American Psychological Association.

*Harris, Grant T., N. Zoe Hilton, and Marnie E. Rice. 1993.
Patients admitted to psychiatric hospital: Presenting problems
and resolution at discharge. *Canadian Journal of Behavioural Science* 25:267–85.

*Harris, John, J. L. T. Birley, and K. W. M. Fulford. 1993. A
proposal to classify happiness as a psychiatric disorder. *British
Journal of Psychiatry* 162:539–42.

*Harrison, Michelle. 1985. *Self-help for premenstrual syndrome.*
New York: Random House.

*Heinrichs, R. Walter. 1993. Schizophrenia and the brain: Condi-
tions for a neuropsychology of madness. *American Psychologist*
48:221–33.

*Herman, Judith. 1988. Review of Self-defeating Personality Disorder. Prepared for *DSM-IV* Work Group on Personality Disorders.

*Hollingshead, August deBelmont, and Fredrick Carl Redlich. 1958. *Social class and mental illness: A community study.* New York: Wiley.

*Houser, Betsy B. 1979. An investigation of the correlation between hormonal levels in males and mood, behavior, and physical discomfort. *Hormones and Behavior* 12:185–97.

Hyler, S., J. B. W. Williams, and R. L. Spitzer. 1982. Reliability in the DSM-III field trials. *Archives of General Psychiatry* 39:1275–78.

Javed, Nayyar. 1994. Panel presentation about *DSM.* Psychologists' Society of Saskatchewan conference. Regina, Sask., Canada. April 28.

*Jensvold, Margaret. 1993. Workplace sexual harassment: The use, misuse, and abuse of psychiatry. *Psychiatric Annals* 23:438–45.

*Jensvold, Margaret, and Ginger Breggin. 1992. The Tailhook of the medical establishment. Press release.

Jensvold, Margaret, and F. Putnam. 1990. Postabuse syndromes in premenstrual syndrome patients and controls. Paper presented at the National Conference of the Association of Women in Psychology. Tempe, Ariz. March.

Jensvold, Margaret, Kathleen Reed, David Jarrett, and Jean Hamilton. 1992. Menstrual cycle-related depressive symptoms treated with variable antidepressant dosage. *Journal of Women's Health* 1:109–15.

Johnson, Barbara. 1993. Pembroke Center lecture, Brown University, December 1.

*Jordan, Judith, et al. 1991. *Women's growth in connection: Writings from the Stone Center.* New York: Guilford.

*Kaminer, Wendy. 1992. *I'm dysfunctional, you're dysfunctional.* Reading, Mass.: Addison-Wesley.

*Kaplan, Marcie. 1983. A woman's view of DSM-III. *American Psychologist* 38:786–97.

Kass, F., R. A. MacKinnon, and R. L. Spitzer. 1986. Masochistic personality: An empirical study. *American Journal of Psychiatry* 143:216–18.

*Kazak, Anne E., Kathryn McCannell, Elizabeth Adkins, Paul Himmelberg, and Janet Grace. 1989. Perception of normality in families: Four samples. *Journal of Family Psychology* 2:277–309.

*Kendall, Kathleen. 1992. Dangerous bodies. In David Farrington and Sandra Walklate, eds., *Offenders and victims: Theory and policy.* British Society of Criminology.

Kessler, R. C., K. A. McGonagle, S. Zhao, C. B. Nelson, M. Hughes, S. Eshleman, H. Wittchen, and K. S. Kendler. 1994. Lifetime and 12-month prevalence of *DSM-III-R* psychiatric disorders in the United States: Results from the National Comorbidity Survey. *Archives of General Psychiatry* 51:8–19.

*****King, D. S.** 1988. Can allergic exposure provoke psychological symptoms? A double-blind test. *Biological Psychiatry* 16:3–19.

*****Kinsbourne, Marcel, and Paula J. Caplan.** 1979. *Children's learning and attention problems.* Boston: Little, Brown.

*****Kirk, Stuart, and Herb Kutchins.** 1992. *The selling of DSM: The rhetoric of science in psychiatry.* New York: Aldine DeGruyter.

*****Kirk, Stuart, and Herb Kutchins.** 1988. Deliberate misdiagnosis in mental health practice. *Social Service Review* 62, 225–37.

*****Kitzinger, Celia.** 1990. Heterosexism in psychology. *The Psychologist.* 3.391–92.

*****Klebanov, Pamela K. and John B. Jemmott.** 1992. Effects of expectations and bodily sensation on self-reports of premenstrual symptoms. *Psychology of Women Quarterly* 16, 289–310.

*****Kleinman, D. L., and L. J. Cohen.** 1991. The decontextualization of mental illness: The portrayal of work in psychiatric drug advertisements. *Social Science and Medicine* 32:867–74.

Klerman, Gerald. 1988. Classification and DSM-III-R. In Armand Nicholi, Jr., ed., *The new Harvard guide to psychiatry.* Cambridge: Harvard University Press, pp. 70–87.

*****Klerman, Gerald L., George E. Vaillant, Robert L. Spitzer, and Robert Michels.** 1984. A debate on *DSM-III. American Journal of Psychiatry* 141:539–42. The * is appropriate here because of Vaillant's comments.

*****Kovel, Joel.** 1988. A critique of DSM-III. *Research in Law, Deviance and Social Control* 9:127–46.

*****Kovel, Joel.** 1980. The American mental health industry. In D. Ingleby, ed., *Critical psychiatry.* New York: Pantheon.

*****Kovel, Joel.** 1978. Things and words: Metapsychology and the historical point of view. *Psychoanalysis and Contemporary Thought* 1:21–88.

*****Kramer, Yale.** 1994. Schizophrenia—and psychiatry's limits. *The Wall Street Journal*, March 9, p. A14.

Kutchins, Herb, and Stuart A. Kirk. In press. *Making diagnoses: DSM and the creation of mental disorder.*

*****Kutchins, Herb, and Stuart A. Kirk.** 1989. DSM-III-R: The conflict over new psychiatric diagnoses. *Health and Social Work*, 91–101.

*Kutchins, Herb, and Stuart A. Kirk. 1988. The business of diagnosis: DSM-III and clinical social work. *Social Work* 33: 215–20.

*Laidlaw, Toni Ann, Cheryl Malmo, and Associates. 1990. *Healing voices: Feminist approaches to therapy with women.* San Francisco: Jossey Bass.

*Laing, R. D. 1967. *The politics of experience.* Baltimore: Penguin.

*Landrine, H. 1989. The politics of personality disorder. *Psychology of Women Quarterly* 13:325–39.

†Landsberg, Michele. 1993. Calling PMS a psychiatric disorder is sheer madness. *Toronto Star*, March 12, p. J1.

*Larkin, June, and Paula J. Caplan. 1992. The gatekeeping process of the DSM. *Canadian Journal of Community Mental Health* 11:17–28.

*Latour, Bruno. 1987. *Science in action: How to follow scientists and engineers through society.* Milton Keynes, England: Open University Press.

†Laurence, Leslie. 1993. Debating classification of PMS. *Connecticut Post*, May 2.

*Lavin, Carl H. 1994. When moods affect safety: Communication in a cockpit means a lot a few miles up. *New York Times*, June 26, p. 18.

*Laws, S., V. Hey, and A. Eagan. 1985. *Seeing red: The politics of pre-menstrual tension.* Dover, N.H.: Hutchinson and Co.

†Lehman, Betsy. 1993. A little revision is creating a big furor. *Boston Globe*, May 10, pp. A1, A16.

*Leo, John. 1994. *Two steps ahead of the thought police.* New York: Simon & Schuster.

*Leo, John. 1985. Battling over masochism. *Time.* December 2, p. 76.

Levene, Marlene. 1992. *Women's experience of self-blame for incestuous abuse: A feminist analysis.* Unpublished doctoral dissertation. University of Toronto.

*Light, Donald. 1980. *Becoming psychiatrists: The professional transformation of self.* New York: Norton.

†Linton, Marilyn. 1993. PMS funding a headache. *Toronto Sun*, March 18, p. 52.

*Lipkowitz, Marvin, and Sudharam Idupuganti. 1985. Diagnosing schizophrenia: Criteria sets and reality. *Hospital and Community Psychiatry* 32:344–45.

*Loring, Marti, and Brian Powell. 1988. Gender, race, and

DSM-III: A study of the objectivity of psychiatric diagnostic behavior. *Journal of Health and Social Behavior* 29:1–22.
*Luborsky, Lester, Paul Crits-Cristoph, Jim Mintz, and Arthur Auerbach. 1988. *Who will benefit from psychotherapy? Predicting therapeutic outcomes.* New York: Basic Books.
*Lunbeck, Elizabeth. 1994. *The psychiatric persuasion: Knowledge, gender, and power in modern America.* Princeton, N.J.: Princeton University Press.
Mack, Avram. 1994. The remedicalization of American psychiatric classification. Undergraduate history thesis. University of Michigan. Ann Arbor.
*Marcus, Lotte. 1991. Therapy junkies. *Mother Jones*, March/April, pp. 60–64.
Marks, Philip, William Seeman, and Deborah Haller. 1974. *The Actuarial use of the MMPI with adolescents and adults.* Baltimore: Williams and Wilkins.
*Marshall, John. 1982. *Madness: An indictment of the mental health care system in Ontario.* Toronto: Ontario Public Services Employees Union.
*Martin, Emily. 1987. *The woman in the body: A cultural analysis of reproduction.* Boston: Beacon.
*Martinez, Julia. 1994. Doctor sues for disability money. *Philadelphia Inquirer.* July 14, p. B01.
*Masson, Jeffrey Moussaieff. 1991. *Final analysis.* Reading, Mass.: Addison-Wesley.
*Masson, Jeffrey Moussaieff. 1988. *Against therapy: Emotional tyranny and the myth of psychological healing.* New York: Atheneum.
*Masson, Jeffrey Moussaieff. 1986. *A dark science: Women, sexuality, and psychiatry in the nineteenth century.* New York: Farrar, Straus and Giroux.
*Masson, Jeffrey Moussaieff. 1984a. *The assault on truth: Freud's suppression of the seduction theory.* New York: Farrar, Straus and Giroux.
*Masson, Jeffrey. 1984b. The persecution and expulsion of Jeffrey Masson as performed by members of the Freudian establishment and reported by Janet Malcolm of *The New Yorker.* *Mother Jones*, December, pp. 34–37, 42–47.
Maxmen, Jerrold. 1985. *The new psychiatry.* New York: Morrow.
*McFarland, Cathy, Michael Ross, and Nancy DeCourville. 1989. Women's theories of menstruation and biases in recall of menstrual symptoms. *Journal of Personality and Social Psychology* 57:522–31.

*McFarlane, Jessica, Carol Lynn Martin, and Tannis MacBeth Williams. 1988. Mood fluctuations: Women versus men and menstrual versus other cycles. *Psychology of Women Quarterly* 12:201–23.

*McGrath, E., G. P. Keita, B. R. Strickland, and N. F. Russo. 1990. *Women and depression: Risk factors and treatment issues.* Washington, D.C.: American Psychological Association.

†McIver, Mary. 1993. Shrink-wrapped. *Homemaker's.* May, 126.

Menstrual stress cited in child abuse case. 1982. New York Times News Service. May 31.

†McMillen, Liz. 1993. Proposal to define premenstrual syndrome as a mental disorder draws fire. *Chronicle of Higher Education*, March 31, A8.

Mental illness, attitudes. 1990. *Globe and Mail*, August 22, p. A14.

*Miedema, Baukje, and Janet M. Stoppard. 1994. "I just needed a rest": Women's experiences of psychiatric hospitalization. *Feminism and Psychology* 4:251–60.

*Miller, Jean Baker. 1984. The development of women's sense of self. *Work in Progress Paper No. 12.* Wellesley, Mass.: Wellesley College, The Stone Center.

Miller, Michael. 1994. Survey sketches new portrait of the mentally ill. *The Wall Street Journal*, January 14, pp. B1, B6.

*Millett, Kate. 1991. *The loony-bin trip.* New York: Touchstone.

Millon, Theodore. 1983. The DSM-III, an insider's perspective. *American Psychologist*, 806–7.

*Mills, Joyce. 1988. Premenstrual syndrome: Symptom, or source of transformation? *Psychological Perspectives* 19:101–10.

*Minow, Martha. 1987. Interpreting rights: An essay for Robert Cover. *The Yale Law Journal* 96:1860–1915.

*Mirowsky, John. 1990. Subjective boundaries and combinations in psychiatric diagnoses. *The Journal of Mind and Behavior*, summer/autumn, p. 411.

*Mirowsky, John, and Catherine Ross. 1989. Psychiatric diagnosis as reified measurement. *Journal of Health and Social Behavior* 30:11–25.

*Mithers, Carol Lynn. 1994. *Therapy gone mad: The true story of hundreds of patients and a generation betrayed.* Reading, Mass.: Addison-Wesley.

Nash, Heather C. 1994. The effect of the presence of Premenstrual Dysphoric Disorder in the DSM-IV on the perception of premenstrual changes. Master's thesis. Connecticut College. New London, Conn.

*Nelkin, Dorothy. 1987. The culture of science journalism. *Society*, September/October, 17–25.

*Nelkin, Dorothy, and Lawrence Tancredi. 1989. *Dangerous diagnostics: The social power of biological information.* New York: Basic Books.

†Ness, Carol. 1993. Premenstrual moods a mental illness? *San Francisco Examiner*, May 20, pp. A1, A16.

Nicholi, Armand M., Jr., ed. 1988. *The new Harvard guide to psychiatry.* Cambridge, Mass.: Belknap.

Nichols, M. 1984. *Family therapy: Concepts and methods.* New York: Gardner.

*Nikelly, Arthur G. 1992. The pleonexic personality: A new provisional personality disorder. *Individual Psychology* 48:253–60.

Nikelly, Arthur G. Drug advertisements and the medicalization of unipolar depression in women. Unpublished paper. University of Illinois. Urbana, Ill.

*Offer, Daniel, and Melvin Sabshin, eds. 1991. *The diversity of normal behavior: Further contributions to normatology.* New York: Basic Books.

*Offer, Daniel, and Melvin, Sabshin. 1966. *Normality: Theoretical and clinical concepts of mental health.* New York: Basic Books.

Orbach, Susie. 1990. *Fat is a feminist issue.* New York: Berkley.

*Orwell, George. 1977. *1984.* San Diego: Harcourt Brace Jovanovich.

*O'Shea, J. A., and S. Porter. 1981. Double-blind study of children with hyperkinetic syndrome. *Journal of Learning Disabilities* 14:189–91, 237.

Othmer, Ekkehard, and Sieglinde Othmer. 1994. *The clinical interview using DSM-IV.* Washington, D.C.: American Psychiatric Association.

Pantony, Kaye Lee, and Paula J. Caplan. 1993. Science vs. conjecture in the *DSM.* Unpublished paper.

*Pantony, Kaye Lee, and Paula J. Caplan. 1991. Delusional Dominating Personality Disorder: A modest proposal for identifying some consequences of rigid masculine socialization. *Canadian Psychology/Psychologie Canadienne* 32:120–33.

Parlee, Mary Brown. 1994. Personal communication. June 17.

Parlee, Mary Brown. 1989. The science and politics of PMS research. Invited address to Association for Women in Psychology. Newport, R.I.

Parlee, Mary Brown. 1982. Changes in moods and activation levels during the menstrual cycle in experimentally naive subjects. *Psychology of Women Quarterly* 7:119–31.

Parlee, Mary Brown. 1978a. Infradian rhythms in moods and activation levels in adult men. Unpublished paper. Barnard College, Columbia University. New York.

*****Parlee, Mary Brown.** 1978b. Mood cycles. *Psychology Today*, April, pp. 82–91.

*****Parlee, Mary Brown.** 1973. The premenstrual syndrome. *Psychological Bulletin* 80:454–65.

†**Pelletier, Francine.** 1993. Les regles de la folie. *Le Devoir*, April 15.

*****Penfold, P. Susan, and Gillian A. Walker.** 1983. *Women and the psychiatric paradox*. Montreal: Eden Press.

*****Pepper-Smith, Robert, and William Harvey.** 1990. Competency assessments in discharge planning and the question of intergenerational justice. *Westminster Affairs* 3:3–5.

*****Perkins, Rachel.** 1991. Therapy for lesbians? The case against. *Feminism and Psychology* 1:325–38.

Perry, Samuel, Allen Frances, and John Clarkin. 1990. *A DSM-III-R casebook of treatment selection*. New York: Brunner/Mazel.

Pichot, P., J. D. Guelfi, and J. Kroll. 1983. French perspectives on DSM-III. In Robert Spitzer, Janet Williams, and Andrew Skodol, eds., *International perspectives on DSM-III*. Washington, D.C.: American Psychiatric Press, pp. 155–73.

Pincus, Harold. 1993. Personal communication. March 12.

Pirie, Marion. 1988. *The promotion of PMS: A sociological investigation of women and the illness role*. Unpublished doctoral dissertation. York University, Toronto.

*****Pirie, Marion, and Lorrie Halliday Smith.** 1992. Coping with PMS: A women's health center has success with a life skills model. *The Canadian Nurse*, December, pp. 24–25, 46.

*****PMS Information and Referral Newsletter**. 1987. Report of June 25 meeting. (Box 363, Station L, Toronto, Ontario M6E 4Z3 Canada)

Pope, Alexander. 1733/1962. An essay on man. In M. H. Abrams, gen. ed., *The Norton anthology of English literature*, Vol. I. New York: W. W. Norton, pp. 1469–76.

*****Professional Staff of the United States–United Kingdom Cross National Project.** 1974. The diagnosis of psychopathology of schizophrenia in New York and London. *Schizophrenia Bulletin* 1:80–102.

*****Psychiatric diagnosis: A mind-expanding book.** *Psychology Today*, November/December, p. 17.

The Psychiatric Times 3 (8). 1986. Special, 1.

Raimy, V. 1950. *Training in clinical psychology.* New York: Prentice Hall.

Randall, David. 1994. Panel presentation about *DSM.* Psychologists' Society of Saskatchewan conference. Regina, Sask., Canada. April 28.

*Rapaport, Elizabeth. 1993. Generalizing gender: Reason and essence in the legal thought of Catharine MacKinnon. In Louise M. Antony and Charlotte Witt, eds., *A mind of one's own: Feminist essays on reason and objectivity.* Boulder, Colo.: Westview Press, pp. 127–43.

*Rawlings, Edna I., and Dianne K. Carter, eds. 1977. *Psychotherapy for women: Treatment toward equality.* Springfield, Ill.: Charles C. Thomas.

Reame, Nancy, John Marshall, and Robert Kelch. 1992. Pulsatile LH secretion in women with premenstrual syndrome (PMS): Evidence for normal neuroregulation of the menstrual cycle. *Psychoneuroendocrinology* 17:205–13.

*Robbins, Joan Hamerman, and Rachel Josefowitz Siegel, eds. 1983. *Women changing therapy: New assessments, values and strategies in feminist therapy.* New York: Haworth.

*Robertson, John, and Louise F. Fitzgerald. 1990. The (mis)-treatment of men: Effects of client gender role and life-style on diagnosis and attribution of pathology. *Journal of Counseling Psychology* 37:3–9.

Robinson, Gail Erlick. 1993. Letter to Allen Frances for APA Committee on Women. April 28.

*Rosenberg, Morris. 1984. A symbolic interactionist view of psychosis. *Journal of Health and Social Behavior* 25:289–302.

*Rosenfield, Sarah. 1982. Sex roles and societal reactions to mental illness: The labeling of "deviant" deviance. *Journal of Health and Social Behavior* 23:18–24.

*Rosenthal, R., and L. Jacobson. 1968. *Pygmalion in the classroom: Teacher expectation and pupils' intellectual development.* New York: Holt, Rinehart, and Winston.

*Rosewater, Lynne Bravo. 1987. A critical analysis of the proposed Self-defeating Personality Disorder. *Journal of Personality Disorders* 1:220–40.

Rosewater, Lynne Bravo. 1985. A critical statement on the proposed diagnosis of masochistic personality disorder. Presented to American Psychiatric Association's Work Group on Revised DSM-III. November 18.

Rossi, A. S. 1974. Physiological and social rhythms: The study of human cyclicity. Special lecture to American Psychological Association. Detroit. May 9.

*Rothblum, Esther D., Laura J. Solomon, and George W. Albee. 1986. A sociopolitical perspective of DSM-III. In Theodore Millon and Gerald L. Klerman, eds., *Contemporary directions in psychopathology: Toward the DSM-IV.* New York: Guilford, pp. 167–89.

*Rothman, David J. 1971. *The discovery of the asylum: Social order and disorder in the New Republic.* Boston: Little, Brown.

Rovner, S. 1987. A new manual for mental disorders. *Washington Post Health,* May 12, p. 8.

*Ruble, Diane. 1977. Premenstrual symptoms: A reinterpretation. *Science* 197:291–92.

*Rush, Florence. 1980. *The best kept secret: Sexual abuse of children.* New York: Prentice-Hall.

*Salk, Hilary. 1993. About Prozac: Listening to women. *Rhode Island Women's Health Collective Newsletter* 12 (4): 5–7.

*Schacht, T. 1985. DSM-III and the politics of truth. *American Psychologist* 40:513–21.

*Schacht, T., and P. E. Nathan. 1977. But is it good for psychologists? Appraisal and status of DSM-III. *American Psychologist* 32:1017–25.

*Schaie, K. Warner. 1993. Ageist language in psychological research. *American Psychologist* 48:49–51.

*Scheff, Thomas J. 1966. *Being mentally ill.* Chicago: Aldine.

*Schmidt, P. J., L. K. Nieman, G. N. Grover, K. L. Muller, G. R. Merriam, and D. R. Rubinow. 1991. Lack of effect of induced menses on symptoms in women with premenstrual syndrome. *New England Journal of Medicine* 324:1174–79.

*Schofield, William. 1964. *Psychotherapy: The purchase of friendship.* Englewood Cliffs, N.J.: Prentice-Hall.

*Schulberg, H. C., and R. W. Manderscheid. 1989. The changing network of mental health service delivery. In C. A. Taube and D. Mechanic, eds., *The future of mental health services research.* Washington, D.C.: U.S. Department of Health and Human Services, pp. 11–22.

*Schwaber, Evelyne. 1983. Psychoanalytic listening and psychic reality. *International Review of Psycho-analysis* 10:379–92.

*Schwartz, Lynn Sharon. 1985. *Disturbances in the field.* New York: Bantam.

Schwartz, Wendy. 1994. Psychiatric diagnostic practice and feminist thought: Bridging the gap between disparate worlds. Dissertation prospectus, unpublished. University of Michigan, Ann Arbor.

Schwartz, Wendy. 1993. The link between masochism and femininity in theory and diagnosis: The call for context. Unpublished paper. University of Michigan, Ann Arbor.

†**Scotton, Lindsay.** 1993 PMS debate: Is it a mental disorder? *Toronto Star*, April 27, pp. B1, B3.

Secker, Barbara. 1994. Women, health care, and the social construction of mental competency. Presented at Women's Health Conference. McMaster University, Hamilton, Ontario, Canada. April 21–24.

†**Segal, Emma F.** 1994. The D.S.M. debate. *New Woman*, March, p. 95.

Seligman, M. E. P. 1988. Why is there so much depression today? The waxing of the individual and the waning of the commons. Paper presented at the American Psychological Association convention. Washington, D.C.

†**Seligmann, Jean, with David Gelman.** 1993. Is it sadness or madness? Psychiatrists clash over how to classify PMS. *Newsweek*, March 15, p. 66.

***Sharkey, Joe.** 1994. *Bedlam: Greed, profiteering, and fraud in a mental health system gone crazy.* New York: Thomas Dunne/St. Martin's.

***Shepard, Marti, and Marjorie Lee.** 1970. *Games analysts play.* New York: Berkley Medallion Books.

***Showalter, Elaine.** 1985. *The female malady: Women, madness, and English culture, 1830–1980.* New York: Pantheon.

Sides, Ann Goodwin. 1993. Personal communication. April 1.

***Siegel, Rachel Josefowitz.** 1993. Between midlife and old age: Never too old to learn. *Women and Therapy* 14:173–85.

***Siegel, Rachel Josefowitz.** 1988. Women's "dependency" in a male-centered value system: Gender-based values regarding dependency and independence. *Women and Therapy* 7:113–23.

***Siegel, Rachel Josefowitz, and Ellen Cole, eds.** 1991. *Jewish women in therapy: Seen but not heard.* New York: Haworth.

***Skrypnek, B. J., and M. Snyder.** 1982. On the self-perpetuating nature of stereotypes about women and men. *Journal of Experimental Social Psychology* 18:277–91.

***Sleek, Scott.** 1994. Could Prozac replace demand for therapy? *American Psychological Association Monitor*, April, p. 28.

†**Socha, Miles.** 1993. PMS designation as psychiatric illness rapped: Protest grows against "oppressive" labelling of some premenstrual syndrome. *Kitchener-Waterloo Record*, March 25, p. F8.

†**Solomon, Alissa.** 1993. Girl crazy: Psychiatry tries to make PMS a mental illness. *The Village Voice*, April 6, pp. 32–33.

***Solomon, Lee A.** 1995. The legal implications of classifying PMS as a mental disorder. *Maryland Law Review 54.*

***Sommer, B.** 1973. The effect of menstration on cognitive and perceptual-motor behavior: A review. *Psychosomatic Medicine 35,* 515–34.

†**Span, Paula.** 1993. Vicious cycle: The politics of periods. *Washington Post,* July 8, pp. C1–C2.

Spitzer, Robert. 1985. Letter to Teresa Bernardez. October 31.

Spitzer, Robert, J.B. Forman, and J. Nee. 1979. DSM-III field trials: I. Initial interrater diagnostic reliability. *American Journal of Psychiatry* 136, 815–77.

Spitzer, Robert, Miriam Gibbon, Andrew Skodol, Janet Williams, and Michael First. 1994. *DSM-IV casebook.* Washington, D.C.: American Psychiatric Association.

Spitzer, Robert, J. Hyler, and J.B. Williams. 1980. Appendix C: Annotated comparative listing of DSM-II and DSM-III. In American Psychiatric Association. *Diagnostic and statistical manual of mental disorders—III.* Washington, D.C. : Author.

Spitzer, Robert, Janet Williams, Miriam Gibbon, and Michael First. 1990 *SCID (Structured Clinical Interview for DSM-III-R).* Washington, D.C. American Psychiatric Association.

Spitzer, Robert, Janet Williams, and A. E. Skodol. 1980. DSM-III: the major achievements and an overview. *American Journal of Psychiatry* 137, 151–64.

***Steinem, Gloria.** 1994. Womb envy, testyria, and breast castration anxiety: Gloria Steinem asks: What if Freud were female? *Ms,* March/April, pp. 48–56.

***Steinem, Gloria.** 1992. *Revolution from within: A book of self-esteem.* Boston: Little, Brown.

†**Stockwood, Kristina.** 1993. Crazy idea: PMS to be classified as mental illness. *Montreal Mirror,* April 15, p. 9.

***Stone, Deborah.** 1989. At risk in the welfare state. *Social Research* 56:591–633.

***Strupp, H. H.** 1986. Psychotherapy: Research, practice, and public policy (How to avoid dead ends). *American Psychologist* 41:120–30.

†**Suh, Mary.** 1993. Severe PMS: Is it mental illness or just normal behavior? *Ms* May/June.

***Szasz, Thomas.** 1994. *Cruel compassion: Psychiatric control of society's unwanted.* New York: John Wiley.

***Szasz, Thomas.** 1970. *The manufacture of madness.* New York: Harper and Row.

*Szasz, Thomas. 1961. *The myth of mental illness: Foundations of a theory of personal conduct.* New York: Delta.

+Tavris, Carol. 1993. You haven't come very far, baby. *Los Angeles Times*, March 4, p. B7.

*Tavris, Carol. 1992. *The mismeasure of woman.* New York: Simon and Schuster.

*Temerlin, Maurice K., and William W. Trousdale. 1969. The social psychology of clinical diagnosis. *Psychotherapy: Theory, Re serach and Practice* 6:24–29.

Tsuang, Ming T., Mauricio Tohen, and Jane M. Murphy. 1988. Psychiatric epidemiology. In Armand M. Nicholi, Jr., ed., *The new Harvard guide to psychiatry.* Cambridge, Mass.: Belknap, pp. 761–79.

Tummon, Ian. 1993. Personal communication, June.

*Tummon, Ian, and Barry Kramer. 1994. Time to discard the diagnosis of premenstrual syndrome? *Journal of the Society of Obstetricians and Gynecologists* 16:1565–70.

*Umbarger, Carter, Andrew Morrison, James Dalsimer, and Peter Breggin. 1962. *College students in a mental hospital: An account of organized social contacts between college volunteers and mental patients in a hospital community.* New York: Grune and Stratton.

*Vice, Janet. 1993. *From patients to persons: The psychiatric critiques of Thomas Szasz, Peter Sedgwick and R. D. Laing.* New York: Peter Lang.

†Vines, Gail. 1993. Have periods, will seek therapy. *New Scientist*, July 31, pp. 12–13.

*Viscott, David. 1972. *The making of a psychiatrist.* New York: Arbor House.

*Walker, Barbara. 1987. *The skeptical feminist: Discovering the virgin, mother, and crone.* San Francisco: Harper and Row.

*Walker, Lenore. 1993. Are personality disorders gender biased? Yes! In S. A. Kirk and S. D. Einbinder, eds., *Controversial issues in mental health.* New York: Allyn and Bacon.

*Walker, Lenore. 1991. Discussion: DDPD: Consequences for the profession of psychology. *Canadian Psychology* 32:137.

*Walker, Lenore. 1987. Inadequacies of the Masochistic Personality Disorder diagnosis for women. *Journal of Personality Disorders* 1:183–89.

*Walker, Lenore. 1986. Masochistic Personality Disorder, take two: A report from the front lines. *Feminist Therapists' Institute Interchange*, January.

*Walker, Lenore. 1984. *Battered woman syndrome.* New York: Springer.

*Walsh, F. 1982. *Normal family processes.* New York: Guilford.

Williams, Janet. 1985. The multiaxial system of DSM-III: Where did it come from and where should it go? II. Empirical studies, innovations, and recommendations. *Archives of General Psychiatry* 42, 181–86.

Williams, Janet, Miriam Gibbon, Michael First, Robert Spitzer, Mark Davies, Jonathan Borus, Mary Howes, John Kane, Harrison Pope, Bruce Rounsaville, and Hans-Ulrich Wittchen. 1992. The structured clinical interview for DSM-III-R (SCID): II. Multisite test-retest reliability. *Archives of General Psychiatry* 49:630–36.

*Wing, J. K., and G. W. Brown. 1970. *Institutionalism and schizophrenia.* Cambridge: Cambridge University Press.

*Wootton, B. 1978. *Social science and social pathology.* Westport, Conn.: Greenwood Press.

*Zimmerman, Mark. 1988. Why are we rushing to publish DSM-IV? *Archives of General Psychiatry* 45:1135–38.

*Zubin, J. 1977–78. But is it good for science? *The Clinical Psychologist* 31:1, 7.

Index

normal and abnormal dichotomy of, 3
research on, 137, 209, 210
symptoms of, 161–165
treatment of, 99, 156
see also Premenstrual Dysphoric Disorder (PMDD)
Problems in living
labeling as mental illness, xvii, 77
medicalization of, xvii
necessity of classifying, 23–26
and seeking therapy, 20
Prozac, 147, 266, 278, 279
Psychiatric News, 233
"Psychiatric survivors," 281, 282, 284
Psychiatrists
M.D. background of, 29
power and influence of, 27–31
Psychoactive Substance Use Disorder, 280
Psychoanalysis, 39, 285
Psychotherapists
ability to help, 20–22
and agreement on diagnosis, 27, 40
effect of suggestion on, 64–68
labeling by, 285
moral questions for, 21–22
offensive attitudes of, 25
see also Patient-therapist relationship
Psychotherapy
defined, xxiii
dependency in, 13–14
industry of, xxiii
negative associations of, 13

reasons for seeking, xvi, 19–20, 23–26
Psychotherapy: The Purchase of Friendship (Schofield), 75
Psychotropic drugs, 16–17, 151, 231, 278
Puberty, normality in, 2

Racism, 50, 62, 191, 280, 284, 318
Racist Personality Disorder, proposal for, 221
Radio shows, 127, 263–266, 293
Randall, David, 281
Rape victims, 86–87
Rapists, 86–87
Reality
defining, 50
in or out of touch with, 5, 45–46, 49–50
Reality-testing model, 49–51
Research
basis of, 26–32
bias in, 49 (*see also* Sexism)
principles in, 20–21
reliability and validity in, 197–202
see also DSM (*Diagnostic and Statistical Manual of Mental Disorders*); *specific editions of DSM; specific disorders*
Resistance Against Psychiatry, 282
Robinson, Gail, 158
Rosenbaum, Jerry, 278
Rosewater, Lynne Bravo, 89, 91, 105
Ross, Catherine, 203
Rubinow, David, 120

Rush, A.John, 137, 138, 238

Sacks, Diane, 164
San Francisco Examiner, 254, 258
Schizophrenia
    diagnosing, 27
    research on, xvii
Schofield, William, 75
Schwaber, Evelyne, 285
Schwartz, Wendy, 208
Scotton, Lindsay, 256
Selective Mutism, 215
Self-Defeating Personality
    Disorder (SDPD),
    168, 177
    criterion for, 79, 91, 101,
        104, 179–180,
        191–192, 205–208
    DSM description of,
        87–88, 90
    as a legal defense, 120–121
    and the media, 121
    misuse and misdiagnosis
        with, 30–31, 80, 104,
        105, 116
    opposition to, 89–90, 94,
        95, 97, 99–121
    in the provisional appen-
        dix, 108, 109, 110, 113
    research for, 102, 103,
        105, 109, 113–114,
        116, 179, 204–205, 206,
        207, 209, 215
    sexism in, 79, 181, 208, 237
    support for, 92–93
    see also Masochistic Per-
        sonality Disorder
        (MPD)
Self-esteem. *See also* Self-
    Defeating Personality
    Disorder (SDPD)
Self-esteem, low, 93

Self-help groups, 47–48,
    73–74, 163
Selling of DSM, The (Kirk &
    Kutchins), xx, 15,
    28–29, 62, 77, 84n, 195
Severino, Sally, 100, 138,
    150, 238
Sex differences
    in abnormality, 6–7
    in anger, 128, 129
    in passivity, 50–51
Sex discrimination, 120–121,
    151
    court case, 120–121,
        208–209
    see also Sexism
Sexism
    in the APA, 169
    in diagnosis, 283
    in the *DSM*, 78–80, 90,
        93–94, 105, 128,
        151–158, 160–167, 179,
        181, 208, 237, 259,
        264, 266
    Freud and, 25, 37–38, 70
    in labeling, 39–40, 97, 441
    in the NIMH, 121
    and normality, 6–7, 78–80
    and sexual abuse, 25,
        37–38
Sexual abuse, 37–38
    in childhood, 37–38,
        63–64
    Freud's view of, 25, 37–38
    use of *DSM* for, 237–238
    victims of, 25, 37–38,
        63–64, 79, 274, 284
Sexual activity, persistent de-
    sire for, 78
Sexual Disorders Not Other-
    wise Specified, 181
Sexual Dysfunction Not

Permission Acknowledgments